WALKING WOMAN
STEP-BY-STEP TO A HEALTHIER HEART

By Harriet Hodgson, BS, MA

Cover design by Jay Highum, Action Graphic Design, Rochester, MN, USA.
Photo source: www.istockphoto.com
Cover photo by Steve Debenport.
Stretching woman photo by Mark Bowden.
Woman power walking photo by Michael Krinke.

What are Readers Saying about *Walking Woman*?

*I intended to start reading **Walking Woman**, but just kept reading and, before I knew it, had read it from beginning to end. It is great – informative, very thorough, humorous at times, personal at times, and beautifully written! In fact, I couldn't put it down. I can personally say that walking with some- one really deepens the bonds of friendship and Harriet Hodgson promotes this beautifully.*

Marcia, Business Owner

*I found **Walking Woman** to be a motivational and educational book to help one get started on a healthier path through walking – no equipment necessary – just a pair of good walking shoes. The excellent medical references that Harriet pro- vides are an added bonus of information on walking to promote better health. I'm inspired to lace up my walking shoes and get moving!*

Jeanine, Statistitian

***Walking Woman** drew me in from the start as a useful resource to changing my life in the easiest way imaginable: walking. This book convinced me that walking can be an exercise program that works for anyone no matter what their athletic ability or personal situation. Its thorough consideration of all of the ele- ments from preparation to equipement to safety and enjoyment on the trail seem to ensure success. All that remains is to grab a friend and take that first step.*

Heidi, Registered Nurse

Whether you are a walker or have a desire to be one, this book is for you. Harriet has words that will inspire you to start walking or keep you walking. I found helpful, healthy tips and recipes for a good diet and fitness. This book is beau- tifuly written with powerful messages and quotes that motivate and inspire. I can't wait for my "spring event" walk.

Amy, Clinical Assistant

WALKING WOMAN
STEP-BY-STEP TO A HEALTHIER HEART

By Harriet Hodgson, BS, MA

www.harriethodgson.com

Thanks to
Sharonne Hayes, MD, FACC for her encouragement
and
Carol Allred of WomenHeart for her helpful suggestions.

Walking is a journey of health and a journey of self.
Harriet Hodgson

Table of Contents

Benefiting from this Book

If you are at risk for heart disease, been diagnosed with it, have suffered a heart attack, recovering from heart surgery, have a sedentary job, a sedentary lifestyle, or want to be fit, this guide is for you. It is divided into two parts, facts and quotes. Part one, walking facts and sources, is the foundation of your fitness program. Part two, a Walking Buddies form, Walking Log pages, and walking-related quotations, is designed to keep you moving.

The guide helps you keep the promise you made to yourself, a promise of self-care and living a healthier life. It is a worthy promise.

Arranged sequentially, the guide begins with making the fitness decision, and moves on quickly to walking benefits, bypassing barriers, getting the right shoes, using a pedometer, warming up, walking safety, staying with your fitness program, and walking after surgery. Since many women have little time for reading these days, I've kept the chapters short and packed them with information. Personal stories bring this information to life. To understand the scope of information, you may wish to speed read part one, go back, and read it a second time for content.

The quotes represent many walking-related topics: stretching, hydration, nutrition, snacks, appearance, aging, body image, attitude, persistence, meditation, nature, environment, weather, friendship, motherhood, and sisterhood. There are 365 quotes in all, one for each day of the year. Read the quotes any way you like, one a day, a page a day, or jump around from page to page.

Some quotes touch the soul, as with Helen Keller's quote about walking with her face towards the sun. Other quotes touch the funny bone, as with Erma Bombeck's quote about not accepting a drink from a urologist. Still others come from government agencies such as the United States Forest Service, which received the comment, "A McDonald's would be nice at trailhead."

Highlight the quotes that appeal to you. You may also jot down a favorite quote on a small piece of paper and tuck it in your pocket. Read the quote while you are walking or give it to a walking buddy. Memorize some of your favorite quotes and say them to yourself while you are walking. One or two meaningful words can be motivating and one quote could become your mantra. Photos of yourself can be motivating as well.

Recent photos of me show a chubby-faced person. Until I reached late middle age I was a thin person and never thought about my weight. Losing weight was a strange concept for me and I wasn't sure how to approach it. One day I found a newspaper drawing of a person with his mouth wide open, tongue hanging out so far his tonsils were visible. I cut out the picture and stuck it on the refrigerator door. Beneath the drawing I wrote, "I have the right to be thin." I even made up a little song about having the right *and the might* to be thin again.

The drawing stayed on the refrigerator for months and I looked at it every time my willpower sagged. Time passed and the drawing became faded, yellow, and so frayed I took it down. The drawing is long gone, yet it remains in my mind, along with the "Don't eat too much" message it conveyed.

If you're anything like me, you need to prepare yourself for the trail ahead. It can be a rocky trail, one that causes you to stumble. The first time I lost weight I was doing well, and then my weight loss stalled. Apparently I had reached a weight loss plateau, a lack of weight loss despite physical activity and healthy eating. Weeks passed and I started to lose weight again. I continued to lose until I hit my target of 120 pounds.

When and if you hit a weight-loss plateau, stop and assess your fitness plan. Have you set realistic goals? Modify them if they aren't realistic. You may also wish to delete some of your goals. Eat less, walk more, and add more physical activity to your days, such as lifting weights. "Don't let a weight-loss plateau lead to an avalanche," Mayo Clinic cautions in a website article. Talk with your physician and/or dietitian if you're unable to get past this plateau.

You and a friend may wish to read the guide together. This gives you opportunities to compare facts, discuss your favorite quotes, and acknowledge your personal weaknesses and strengths. Your strengths may help a friend to reach her fitness goal. Similarly, her strengths may help you reach yours. Best of all, you can approach fitness and staying fit together.

This guide may be a good choice for your book club. In addition to discussing some of its points, you may discuss how you stay fit, and how you care for your heart. Members may talk about what they do to care for their health. You may also discuss healthy weight maintenance, a concern that many women share. This guide cites my weight loss progress and I want to make something clear to you. I am not trying to become as thin as a Barbie doll; I'm trying to be slender and fit for my age. (Notice that I didn't use the word skinny.)

Walking Woman is my fitness companion and, hopefully, it will become yours. Within these pages you will find information, motivation, and laughter. You may also find yourself. Fact-by-fact, quote-by-quote, step by-step, this book helps you walk your way better health. Put down that television remote and get going!

Resource

1. Mayo Clinic website, www.mayoclinic.com, "Getting Past a Weight-Loss Plateau."

Introduction

The idea for **Walking Woman** came from life experience. About eight years ago, when I had my annual physical exam, medical tests showed a slightly elevated blood sugar. To reduce the burden on my heart keep me from developing type two diabetes like my mother, my doctor asked me to lose weight. Her advice, and getting on the scale, were a health wake-up call.

"The next time you see me I will be thinner," I promised.

I joined a health club, walked on a treadmill, and walked in my neighborhood. Though my weight dropped with agonizing slowness, thankfully it dropped. A year later I was 25 pounds lighter. Losing so much weight changed my appearance and when I returned for my next yearly exam the nurses barely recognized me. "Wow!" one sad, looking me up and down. My doctor also had a wow reaction.

"You did everything I asked," she said, "and it shows."

Years passed, and I continued to maintain a weight of 120 pounds or so, within the normal range for a small-boned person who is five feet, five inches tall. This weight was also within a normal Body Mass Index (BMI) range, a calculation that helps you determine the percentage of fat in relation to height, build and age.

My pedometer became an extra appendage and I walked 10,000 steps a day. One day I surprised myself and walked 18,000 steps, too far, and I ached for a long time afterwards. As my walking program continued, I used up three pedometers. One, a "freebie," fell apart and two stopped working after they dropped to the ground. Still, I kept walking.

I also lowered my consumption of meat by a third and replaced the meat with fruits and vegetables, which I love. Vegetables became such a large part of my diet I expected broccoli to sprout from my ears and my skin to develop a greenish tinge. My fitness program came to a sudden halt when tragedy struck my family.

In 2007 my elder daughter died from the injuries she received in a car crash. Two days later, on the same weekend, my father-in-law succumbed to pneumonia. Eight weeks after that my brother, and only sibling, died of a heart attack. He had been battling cancer and, though he survived the treatment, his heart did not. Grieving for family members made my husband and me tired and listless. We sat on the couch and sobbed for weeks.

"I don't think we will ever be happy again," I commented.

Our tears slowly abated and the day came when we arose from the couch and went for a walk in the neighborhood. Moving felt good after being inactive so long. We continued to walk in the neighborhood, about twice a week, until tragedy struck again. In the fall of the same year, my twin grandchildren's father died from the injuries he received in another car crash. Losing four family members within nine months was unbelievable and we were paralysed with grief.

"Hollywood would reject this plot," a friend commented. "It's too emotional." I agreed with her.

Their father's death made our grandchildren orphans and my husband and me GRGs, an acronym for grandparents raising grandchildren. The twins moved in with us when they were 15 ½ years old. Our quiet house became a noisy house, filled with the sounds of drum beats, trumpet "runs," choir practice, blaring rock music, running footsteps, and teenage laughter. Having teens in the house again was a blessing, but caring for them while grieving proved to be the biggest challenge of my life.

Would I survive such tragedy? Since I've always had normal blood pressure, I never worried about having it checked. Stress changed all that. When I had my annual physical exam my blood pressure was 205 over something (I can't remember the second number). All I know is that it was at a dangerous level. This surprised me because I felt the same as I usually felt and hadn't noticed any health changes. No wonder high blood pressure is called the silent killer.

According to the *Harvard Heart Letter* stress constricts blood vessels, speeds heart beats, and makes the heart and blood vessels reactive to more stress. Certainly, my life was filled with stressful experiences: appearing in court, submitting legal/financial documents, finding our daughter's financial assets, loving, protecting, and caring for grandchildren, clearing out our daughter's house, and putting it up for sale. The stress was never-ending.

If I had a stress meter with settings spaced like clock numbers, and a clock hand that pointed to them, the progression would look like something like this.

START: Grieving for multiple losses.

ARROW HIGHER: Lifestyle change and raising grandchildren.

ARROW HIGHER: Daughter's unpaid emergency surgery bill, more than a quarter of a million dollars.

ARROW HIGHER: Finishing lower level of daughter's home.

ARROW HIGHER: Lower level floods due to faulty sump pump valve.

ARROW HIGHER: Repairing lower level.

ARROW HIGHER: Lower level floods a second time.

ARROW HIGHER: Repairing lower level again.

STILL HIGHER: Clearing out daughter's house, which took a year.

DANGEROUSLY HIGH: Daughter's home on market for two years and broken into once. Thankfully, the home wasn't damaged.

HIGHEST SETTING: Diagnosis of high blood pressure and risk of heart disease.

People respond differently to stress, notes a WebMD article, "Heart Disease and Stress." As the article reports, "Chronic stress exposes your body to unhealthy, persistently elevated levels of stress hormones like adrenaline and cortisol." Common stressors include the death of a loved one, death of a friend, work overload, and legal problems, the article continues.

I experienced all of these stressors and more.

The relationship between stress and heart disease is still fuzzy, so researchers continue to study it. Stress can cause blood pressure to spike temporarily, according to a Mayo Clinic website article. "Adding up short-term stress-related spikes in your blood pressure may put you at risk for developing long-term high blood pressure," the article points out. When I read this sentence I felt like it was describing me.

Before the twins (one boy, one girl) moved in with us, we ate light meals – fish, lean meat or chicken, vegetables or salad for dinner. But my granddaughter was on the gymnastics team, my grandson was in the marching band, and was on the track team briefly. Like most teenagers the twins were always hungry. I prepared larger meals, with protein, starch, vegetable, salad, and dessert if the twins wanted it. Most of the time I ate the same meals they ate and, consequently, I piled on the pounds. Of course, I should have fixed separate meals for us, but at the end of the day, I was just too tired.

Physical activity was the last thing on my "To Do" list. I still wanted to write, however. Some friends thought I would have to give up writing in order to care for my grandkids. Giving up the career I loved would feel like another death in the family and it would be mine. The only solution I could think of was to get up earlier. At 4:45 a.m. I stumbled out of bed, bundled myself in a robe, and wrote for an hour before breakfast. I resumed writing after the twins went to school.

Both of them graduated from high school with honors, received scholarships, and left for college, my grandson to a Minnesota state university, my granddaughter to a small private college in Iowa. After they left I began to walk more. Though I didn't walk daily, I walked regularly, at least three times a week, and I was proud of myself. But I could tell my hips were getting creaky. During my annual physical exam I told my doctor about my painful right hip. She thought I had arthritis, ordered x-rays, and they revealed two arthritic hips, not one. My right hip was injected to relieve pain, but the relief lasted only a month.

To complicate matters, I have a heart murmur, a souvenir of childhood Scarlet Fever. I also take two medications to control high blood pressure. These medications slow my heart rate and I can't walk very fast. When added together these factors – blood pressure medicine, heart murmur, arthritic hips, grieving, and caregiving – walking was difficult. Sometimes my right hip hurt enough to prohibit me from walking distances. Yet on other days my hip felt fine and the pain changes were confusing. But one thing was all too clear.

After all of my efforts, all of my dark days, all of my challenges, I was back where I started, 20 pounds overweight.

Several months after my yearly physical I fractured a bone in my foot. Somehow, I hit my arch on the corner of a cupboard. "Ouch!" I exclaimed aloud. "That really hurt." A week later, my foot began to throb and the pain was so intense I went to the hospital emergency room (ER). Actually, it was a Trauma Center, which has a larger staff than an emergency room and more diagnostic equipment. The on-call physician gave me a prescription for a painkiller, told me to stay off my feet, and use crutches. Good advice, but since I couldn't manage the crutches, or stay off my feet in a house with two sets of stairs, it took three months for the fracture to heal.

Valid as these factors were, they were still excuses for not getting regular physical activity. The time had come to break out of the fog, wake up, and take back responsibility for my health. So I dusted off my willpower and returned to my walking program again. I started slowly, walking around each grocery store aisle four times, something that caught the eyes of an employee, who stared at me each time I passed her. I felt like her eyes were boring holes in my back.

"Can I help you?" she asked worriedly. (I think she thought I was demented.)

"No thanks," I replied. I'm getting my daily exercise." She nodded, smiled and walked away.

Now my goal is to walk a half hour each day and I'm meeting this goal. Because stepping on a scale makes me nervous, I use the jeans weight test. When my jeans are tight I've had extra salt, extra food, or less physical activity. Thankfully, I am making progress and jeans that used to feel tight now feel loose. Hooray!

Life has its surprises, both bad and good. When I was deleting old computer files I came across this manuscript. I started it years ago and never finished it. Since the concept was still valid, I made a list of what needed to be done, and worked on each task. Despite years of writing experience, getting back into the manuscript, its purpose, organization, and flow, was a challenge, and it took me several months. But I did it and I'm glad. *Walking Woman* is the book I needed then and it's the book I need now.

My story could almost be every woman's story.

In fact, every woman has a story and yours may be similar to mine, a story of good intentions, successes, failures, diversions, caregiving, crises, illness, and normal aging. Yet hope is not lost. Walking is the easiest and cheapest form of physical activity, and that's why it is the focus of this book. I have focused on women because women's health continues is a top medical issue. Too many women are living with heart disease.

Heart attack is the number one killer of women, according to the American Heart Association. Did you know women's symptoms differ from men's? Men's symptoms include shortness of breath, feeling weak, unusual fatigue, cold sweats, and dizziness. Women's symptoms include shortness of breath and subtle signs as well, things like disturbed sleep, unusual fatigue, indigestion, and anxiety. As the American Heart Association explains, "Women often chalk up the symptoms to less life-threatening conditions like acid reflux, the flu or normal aging."

This sentence grabbed my attention and I hope it grabs yours. Chronic medical problems may mask the symptoms of heart attack. Despite shoulder pain, a woman who has asthma may attribute her breathing difficulties to an asthma attack, not a heart attack, ignore the symptoms, and go to bed and rest. Unfortunately, this can delay the diagnosis, proper treatment, and damage her heart. Scary as heart disease is, you can do something about it.

The American Heart Association says just 30 minutes of physical activity a day can help to reduce the risk of heart disease. ***Walking Woman*** supports the organization's motto, "Walk more. Eat better. Live a longer, healthier life." We can turn this motto into action. Women need to stay connected with each other. Together, we can lose extra pounds, reach a healthy weight, and maintain this weight. I'm a grandmother and have made a fitness promise to myself: *I will walk a half hour for heart health today and all my tomorrows.*

Will you make this promise? Please join me on this walking journey, a journey of health and a journey of self.

Resources

1. Harvard University website, www.health.harvard.edu/press, "Stress and Heart Disease."
2. WebMD website, www.webmd.com, "Heart Disease and Stress."
3. Mayo Clinic website, www.mayoclinic.com, "High Blood Pressure (Hypertension)."

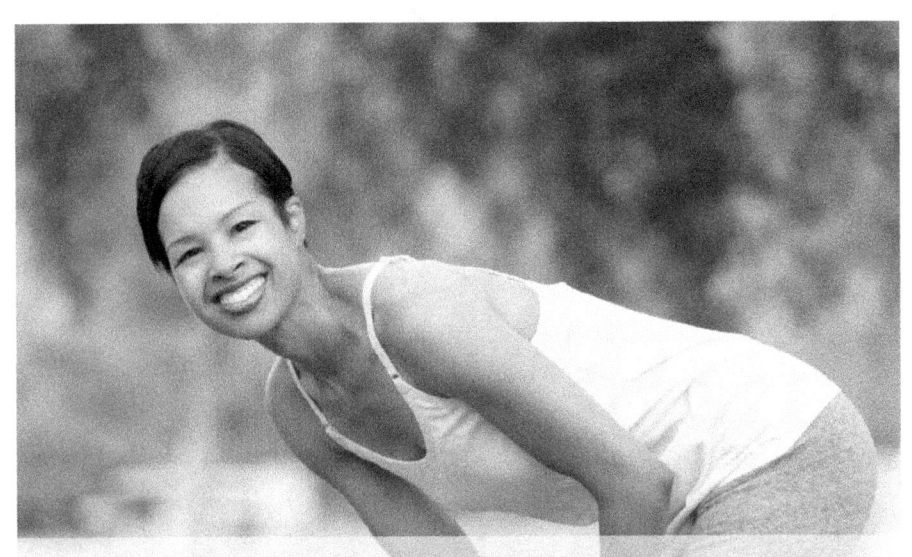

WALKING FACTS:
YOUR FITNESS FOUNDATION

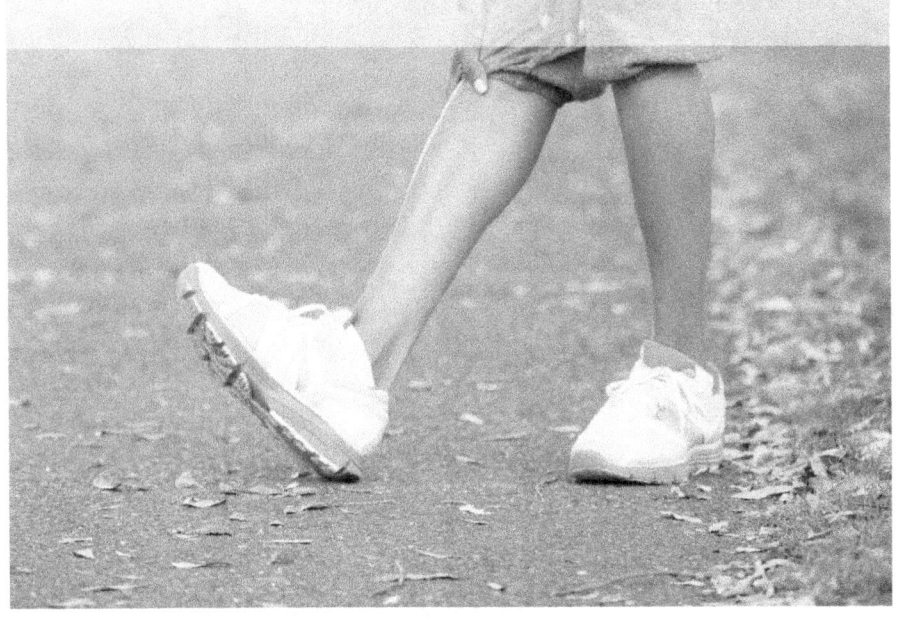

Chapter 1

The Fitness Decision

Fitness isn't a sometime decision; it is a lifetime decision. Starting a fitness program is easy, but as time passes, it may become harder. The fast, hectic, noisy pace of modern life makes it difficult to stay on the fitness path. Yet with determination and planning, you can do it. Walk for your health and all the people who care about you. From experience, I can tell you regular walking is energizing and makes you feel better.

Make walking part of your daily routine. If you're a new mother, you may walk to lose extra tummy weight. If you're the mother of young children, you may walk to have the stamina to keep up with them. If you're a grandmother you may walk because you want to see your grandchildren grow and mature. If you're an experienced grandmother like me, you may walk for better health so you can be at your grandchildren's college graduations.

If you're a woman you walk because you're health-conscious and want to take good care of yourself. That is a worthy goal and you are worthy of it.

But the fitness path isn't a perfect path and there will probably be times when you stray. You may not walk for a week or more. At a wedding reception you may "pig out" at the buffet table and feel awful afterwards. Walking may be impossible because you're at a week-long conference and sitting for hours each day. Circumstances like these aren't the end of your fitness program. Just as a child gets back on a bike after a fall, you get back to your fitness program. You put on your shoes and walk.

Years ago a Rochester, Minnesota nun made the fitness decision for herself. Franciscan sister Vera Klinkhammer decided to walk daily for health and her story is detailed in a *Post-Bulletin* article, "Aging Well 101." Raised on a farm, she was used to regular physical activity and, as a trained nurse, understood the health benefits of it. While she was living at St. Marys Hospital, a Catholic institution and part of Mayo Clinic, the sister walked the hallways each day. She walked and walked and walked. Hospital staff, patients, and visitors were used to seeing her, so used to it that Mayo Clinic wondered how far she walked, and asked her to wear a pedometer for a day.

At the end of the day the sister had walked an astonishing 12 miles! Multiply this distance by the 72 years she lived at the hospital, and she walked nearly half a million miles. Today, at age 101, she is still walking and sharing her advice for longevity, "Just keep going." She thinks people sit too much, according to the article, and that is one reason why she continues to walk. The article quotes the sister as saying she is grateful for each day, her wonderful life, her good health, her functioning senses, and the ability to take care of herself.

A photo of her walking at Assissi Heights, also part of Mayo Clinic, was published with the newspaper article. I studied the photo carefully. Though she is 101 years old, the sister looks like she is in her mid-50s. Sister Klinkhammer is a living example of the health benefits of a walking program and sticking with it.

Making the fitness decision is easier than living it, for staying active requires ongoing effort and re-commitment. You must make the fitness pledge each day. As the sister's story shows, daily walking can help to prolong your life. How can you stay active? You may turn to the Internet first. There is lots of information on the Internet, but you have to sort through it, and figure out what is reliable and what is not. This takes time. Before you become a regular website visitor, join an online community, or subscribe to anything, you need to answer 10 questions.

1. Who pays the bills?
2. Who manages the website?
3. What does the "About Us" section say about the business, organization, or person?
4. Who writes for the website?
5. Are these authors qualified?
6. What else have these authors written?
7. Are the artices evidence-based, purely anecdotal, or just plain false?
8. Is the information current?
9. What do reviews say about the website?
10. Does the website want to help me or just sell me stuff?

While you're surfing the Internet, be wary of pop-up ads and wild claims. Things that sound too good to be true are probably false. Also be wary of magic pills that promise rapid weight loss. The best way to attain and maintain a healthy weight is to eat sensibly and get regular physical activity. Check with your doctor before you start a walking program.

Learn more about the risks of heart disease. Go to www.womenheart.org, click on resources, and download a helpful brochure,

"Get Smart About Your Heart." As the brochure notes, "By adopting heart healthy habits you can lower your risk of heart disease significantly." Make walking one of your habits and your family's habits, something that happens each and every day.

Across the country, in large cities and small towns, women are walking. They have discovered that walking with other women is empowering. Some groups are large, some are small, and some are just two friends walking together. Though the size of the group doesn't matter, daily physical activity does, and it matters a lot.

Personally, I think staying in touch with other women who are living with heart disease or at risk for it, matters as well. Woman-to-woman, experience-to-experience, we can help each other. At this age and stage of life I'm able to look at my journey through a long-distance lens and it has taught me a stunning truth: Walking helps me discover new things about myself. You will make these discoveries too.

Resource

1.   Hansel, Jeff. "Aging Well 101: Rochester Sister has the Right Recipe," *Post-Bulletin*, February 25, 2013, p. C-1.

Chapter 2

Why Should You Walk?

Women want to be healthy. Every day we get up with good intentions. We're going to buy healthy food, fix healthy meals, be physically active, and make time for ourselves. All too often, however, our good intentions are diverted. Once we're diverted, it is easy stay that way. Instead of putting our health first, we put it last, after everything else is done.

Maybe that's because nature programmed us to be nurturers. The increasing demands of nurturing can push us off the fitness path and it can be hard to get back on again. Are too many responsibilities keeping you from caring for yourself? Do you neglect your health because you think self-care is selfish? Have you given up on fitness because you're overweight? Are your extra pounds creeping towards obesity? Is shortness of breath a problem for you?

Your health may be at risk if you answered "yes" to any of these questions. That's the bad news. The good news is that you can change. Indeed, you must change. You must care for yourself so you can care for others.

Print and television media recognize this fact. Pick up any woman's magazine or newspaper and you'll find articles about women's health. Countless women's health articles are posted on the Internet. Television specials focus on specific health issues, such as breast cancer and menopause and infertility. Despite this media blitz, many women still don't take care of themselves. Information isn't the problem, so what is?

One problem is motivation. Even seasoned athletes need motivation to stick to a fitness routine. In order to maintain a fitness program you need to be motivated. What's more, you need to stay motivated, week after week, month after month, year after year. Lack of information, and even misinformation, may be problems as well. It's hard to believe that something as simple as walking can have so many benefits. Why should you walk? There are many reasons and each one impacts your well-being.

- Walking is easy and you know how to do it.
- Walking doesn't require lots of equipment.
- Walking is suitable for all ages (unless you have a medical problem).
- Walking is something you can do alone and with others.
- Walking is a way to cope with stress.
- Walking can be a form of meditation.
- Walking leads to personal discoveries.
- Walking is weight-bearing physical activity; your body is "carrying" your weight.
- Walking increases your stamina.
- Walking helps you reach and maintain a healthy weight.
- Walking can help to prevent heart disease.
- Walking can help you recover from heart surgery. (Chapter 11 has more information on this topic.)

Why Should You Walk?

Your heart is a pump. It isn't an ordinary pump, it is living one, and so efficient it pushes about 2,000 gallons of blood around your body every day. The heart has two sides, left and right, and each side has two chambers. Four one-way valves keep the blood going in the right direction and prevent it from flowing backwards.

Brisk walking for 30 or more minutes five days a week can cut your risk of heart disease by 40 percent, according to Beth Israel Deaconess Medical Center, an affiliate of Harvard Medical School. Walking briskly increases your heart rate and blood circulation. In short, brisk walking makes your heart more efficient and delivers more oxygen to your organs.

A Mayo Clinic website article lists some of the benefits of walking and they include reducing the risk of heart attack, managing blood pressure, managing diabetes, building strength and stamina. All are good reasons to have a regular walking program. Walking can lift your spirits and after a brisk walk life seems brighter.

Walking has another benefit for me. If I'm stuck on a title, paragraph, or searching for a word, I take a walk. Sometimes I walk around the perimeter of a discount store and other times I walk in my neighborhood. During my walk I ignore writing and focus my attention on my environment. I observe people, seasonal changes, watch for birds, and say hello to neighbors. Logically, you would think putting writing out of my mind would work against me. Just the opposite happens. At the end of the walk, the solution to my writing problem appears in my mind like magic.

Older women, and I'm one of them, may not be as steady on their feet as they used to be. If you have a balance problem while walking, instead of looking down at your feet or the sidewalk, look ahead and focus on a distant object, such as a street light. This should steady your balance. You may also link arms with another person or use a walking stick. Some of my family members have made walking sticks from tree branches. Metal sticks are also available from sports stores.

Adults are role models for children, so ask your kids, grandkids, nieces, nephews , and neighbors to walk with you. Make walking fun. Try backwards walking, race walking, baby steps, side steps, twirling steps, and duck steps. Walking races may be something family members would enjoy. When your motivation lags (and it probably will) read the facts section again. You are a woman and worthy of self-care. Keep walking!

Resources

1. Beth Israel Deaconess Medical Center website, www.bidmc.org, "Walking is Good for Your Heart."
2. WebMD website, www.webmd.com, "Heart Disease Health Center."
3. *Heart Surgery and You: A Guide for Teens.* Rochester, MN: Mayo Press, 1996, p. 4-5.
4. Mayo Clinic website, www.mayoclinic.com, "Walking: Trim Your Waistline, Improve Your Health."
5. Mayo Clinic staff, "Defining Exercise," *Mayo Clinic Health Letter,* January 2013, p. 5.

Chapter 3

Bypassing All Those Barriers

Let's be honest. We face many walking barriers: cramps, worry about being injured, actual injury, creaky joints, chronic disease, such as asthma, odd work hours, overtime, poor sleep, low self-esteem, no support system, lack of funds, crises, caregiving tasks, time constraints, balance problems, and aging. Sure, these barriers are daunting, but you can overcome all of them.

Get a physical. If you haven't had a physical exam in years, now is the time to get one. Pay attention to your numbers: cholesterol levels (good and bad), triglycerides, blood pressure, fasting glucose, Body Mass Index (BMI) and waist circumference. Ask your doctor to explain these numbers if you don't understand them. You may also request printed information. Most important, ask your doctor if it is safe to start a walking program. Do not start a program without his or her go-ahead. Does your doctor have any special advice for you?

Start slowly. Though walking is the easiest form of physical activity, that doesn't mean you start out with a 10-mile hike. You may start by walking around the block for a week. The next week you walk two blocks, and so on, gradually increasing the distance, until walking is part of each day. Over time, you will feel a difference in your body and have more stamina. When you reach this point, even though you may be tempted to give up, don't succumb to this temptation, and keep walking.

Add more steps. Parking at the back of the lot is one way to add them. Take the stairs instead of the elevator. Walk the city skyways that connect downtown buildings. Walking meetings – discussions held while walking – is another way to add steps. This suggestion comes from Mayo Clinic's former Action on Obesity Task Force, which also suggested wearing a special tag, "Walking meeting in progress." During bad weather I add steps by walking around the center island in my kitchen. Thirty times around equals 1,000 steps and I watch television while I'm walking. Walking around the kitchen island is boring, but at least I'm moving.

Vary your routine. Like many women, I used to pile items at the bottom of the stairs and take them up all at once to save steps. I don't do this anymore. Though I still pile items at the bottom of the stairs, I take them upstairs separately to get extra steps. Changing my walking place and route also keeps walking interesting. Walking in different cities is something I enjoy because I can observe different architectural, landscaping, and decorating styles.

Use public places and spaces. Walk the city park trails, around an indoor mall, do laps in discount stores, or grocery store aisles. Your city or town may have walking trails. The American Heart Association has established walking paths across America. To find the ones nearest you, visit www.startwalkingnow.org/start_walking_paths.jsp.

People often walk inside malls because it's free, they are sheltered from the elements, and are on a flat surface. A group of women walked in the local mall regularly. While I admired their perseverance, I didn't admire the conclusion of their daily walks, a coffee break that included giant cinnamon buns. Later I learned each bun contained about 1,200 calories.

Move in spurts. Mayo Clinic, in a website article, "Barriers to Fitness: Overcoming Common Challenges," says short, 10-minute spurts of physical activity can be beneficial. The spurt system is a useful approach for people like me who have a sedentary job. I use the spurt system and love it. Over time, small spurts can have a big impact on your health. When I'm writing I try to take a stretching break every 15-25 minutes. This wakes up my mind and keeps me from getting stiff.

Try theme walking. This helps to keep physical activity interesting. Look for birds one day, cloud formations the next, your favorite color, and a specific brand of car. Plan destination walks, treks to historic buildings, public art, and so-called "pocket parks," those small green spaces that soften a city's hardscapes. A newspaper article about pocket parks made me aware of this term, and the many green spaces hidden amidst the buildings in my city. Now, whenever I'm in a different city or town, I look for these green areas.

Take advantage of incentives. McDonald's has given away thousands of free pedometers, a way to foster walking in customers of all ages. Other businesses and organizations give away free water bottles, sun visors, caps, booklets, reflective bands, free cooking demonstrations, and discount coupons. You may as well take advantage of these incentives. While you're at it, give yourself a prize after you reach a major health goal.

Train for hiking. Years ago, my husband and I went to Peru with family members. Our schedule included visiting Machu Picchu, a 15th century Inca city some 7,970 feet above sea level. To prepare myself for the altitude I trained on a stationary bike for months. My training worked. I didn't have any breathing difficulties, enjoyed walking around the ancient stone city, and hiked the Inca Trail with family members. Our goal was an Inca gate. While other family members reached the gte, I did not. I have a fear of heights and, as I climbed higher, the trail became narrower – dangerously narrow.

One misstep and I could stumble, roll down the mountain head over heels, hitting rocks and cacti along the way, until I reached the train station far below. This thought stopped me in my tracks and I burst into tears. I turned around, sat down, and grabbed onto a twig pertruding from the dirt mountainside. Above me, hikers were coming down the trail, and I could hear their clunking walking sticks and conversation long before they reached me.

Every one asked the same question: "Agua señora?" I didn't want water, I wanted a wider trail, a sturdy railing, and level ground.

Slowly, carefully, tearfully, I made my way back down the trail, and reached the meadow where it began. According to my sister-in-law I had come within a few feet of the gate. Even if you have a fear like me, training for a hike is common sense. You may train on a treadmill, walk community trails, or cross-train by combining different kinds of physical activities, such as using a stationary bike, treadmill, and lifting weights. If you don't have weights you can lift cans of food or household items.

Change your walking type. Mindful walking – being acutely aware of your body and environment – is a logical follow-up to theme walking. Nordic Walking with trekking poles may also interest you. According to the *Arthritis Today* website, this walking helps to burn more calories. High-energy walking, also called race walking, is something else you may wish to try. With race walking, the advancing leg is straight, and you walk so fast you never lose contact with the ground. Eventually you may work up to alternate walking and running. Of all of these walking types, mindful walking is my favorite because it's something I can easily do at my age.

Make walking a spiritual experience. You can make each walk a meditation. Similar to mindful walking, walking meditation is usually done outdoors, though it can be done indoors. Kelly McGonigal, PhD details the approach in a *Psychology Today* website article. You start by walking fast enough to increase your heart rate slight. Next you focus your attention on your breathing and your feet hitting the ground. "Shift to a state of open awareness for anywhere from 1-5 minutes," McGonigal advises. Don't daydream, however. Some people use a mantra, a word they say with each step. Walking meditations may be done alone or in a group. With practice, you learn to calm yourself and the random thoughts that come to mind.

Keep a walking log. This has helped some women stay on the fitness path and may help you. It's also fun to look back and see your walking journey. Personally, I like to walk with to someone I can talk to easily, a relative, friend or my husband. That doesn't mean my husband and I talk all the time, however. Sometimes we walk in the neighborhood and don't say a word; we simply enjoy each other's company. Instead of a written log, you may keep a walking log on the Internet, and download free maps that track your accrued mileage. You will find addresses for these logs and maps in the chapter about websites.

Monitor your eating. Track your intake in a food diary or on one of the many websites available, some free and some not, such as www.caloriecount.com. Monitoring was easy for me because I ate Cheerios for breakfast and lunch for weeks. But I must admit, there were times when I felt like a walking Cheerio and, instead of cereal, ate lean meat, vegetable soup, or cottage cheese and fruit for lunch. Before I eat anything I remind myself of my goals to eat less sugar, cook with olive oil, avoid fatty foods, steer clear of salt, and eat normal servings.

Adapt to weather changes. When the temperature plunges, pelting raindrops are falling, and blowing snow clouds the sky, chances are you feel less like walking. Still, you need to keep moving. Bundle up, dress in layers, and continue to walk outdoors, if possible. Radio and television stations in my community tell parents to cover their children's faces when the wind chill is dangerously low and would freeze flesh. Icy sidewalks and fierce windchills prevent me from walking outdoors in the winter. That's why I walk in megastores, malls, and grocery stores.

Reward Yourself. Set attainable goals and reward yourself when you reach them. For example, your goal may be to walk 20 minutes a day for one month. When you reach this goal you may reward yourself with a new t-shirt or the ice cream cone you craved so much. Reading a good mystery is one of my rewards. What are yours? Rewarding yourself every so often fuels your fitness motivation.

Resource

6. McGonigal, Kelly, "Walking Meditation: The Perfect 10-Minute Willpower Boost," *Psychology Today* website, www.psychology.com.

Chapter 4

Stretching for Flexibility

Stretching is good any time. Doing it before you walk helps to prevent leg and foot cramps. According to the *California Walking Kit Training Manual*, you should never bounce or stretch rapidly. Stretches should be held for 15-20 seconds. Don't hold your breath while you stretch; just breathe normally. Above all, don't fall for the idea that pain equals gain because it is false.

A Mayo Clinic website article says stretching is not a warm-up. In fact, you should prepare to stretch before you do it. "Warm-up with light walking, jogging or biking at low intensity for five to 10 minutes," the clinic advises. Walking in place for a few minutes also prepares you for a walk. One more piece of advice from Mayo: "Keep up with your stretching." Here are some stretches to try.

- **The wake-up stretch**. After sleeping animals and humans stretch instinctively. Stretch your arms above your head as if you were waking up in the morning. Continue to stretch, reaching as high as you can, and hold this position for 20 seconds, more if you can do it.

- **Going in circles.** Swing your arms in circles. Go forwards first and then backwards. If you have shoulder problems or shoulder socket problems you may wish to eliminate this stretch.

- **Leg stretch**. This is an old-fashioned stretch, but it's still a good one. Bend over and touch your knees without bending your legs. Do this 10 times. I ued to teach kindergarten and asked my students to do this stretch when they were wiggly. To my astonishment, I discovered that some children couldn't touch their toes without bending their knees. I know this story sounds false, but I can assure you that it is true. Apparently I was in better condition than some of my students.

- **Doing the Sidestep**. Stand normally, with your arms raised to shoulder height. Using one leg, take a step sideways, extending your leg as far as possible. Repeat with the other leg. You will feel this stretch in your thighs.

- **Making curves.** I learned this stretch in a college unit about modern dance. Stretch each arm over your head in an arc. Hold this position for 15-20 seconds. Repeat with your other arm. You will feel this stretch in your torso.

- **Waist twisting.** Stand with your feet slightly apart. Put your hands on your waist and twist from side to side without moving your feet. I like this stretch because it's easy and I feel it in my waist and thighs. You may also do this stretching exercise with your arms at shoulder length, twisting them in circles as you twist your body.

- **Quadriceps stretch.** Bend one leg backwards, grasp your foot and hold this position for 20 seconds. Repeat with the other foot. Stop if you get a cramp in your leg or legs.

- **Body pointing.** Get on your hands and knees. Reach your left arm out straight in front of you and stretch your left leg out straight behind you. Repeat with your other arm and leg, holding this position for 30 seconds. Arthritis prevents me from doing this stretch, but you may be agile enough to do it.

- **Chair hold.** Hold onto a chair. Press one heel onto the floor and push down to stretch your calf. Hold this position for one minute. Repeat with other heel. This is one of the most helpful stretches I do. If I get a leg or foot cramp in the middle of the night, I get up, hold onto the bed, and do this stretch until the cramp goes away.
- **Torso stretches.** This stretching and flexibility exercise comes from the American Heart Association (AHA). Sit in a chair with your feet flat on the floor. Link your hands behind your head and twist your body from side to side. You will find more torso stretches on the AHA website.
- **Opposite stretches.** Sit on the floor or ground, with your legs slightly apart. Touch your right hand to your left foot, and then touch your left hand to your right foot. Hold this position for several seconds and repeat.
- **Foot stretches.** You may be surprised to learn that foot stretching helps you. One stretch is to pick up a washcloth with your toes. Do this with both feet. Heel and toe risers are another stretching exercise for your feet. Stand on the tips of your toes and hold this position. Stand on your heels and hold this position as well. Finally, extend each leg and pull your toes towards you. These foot stretches strengthen your feet, according to Mayo Clinic.

The American College of Sports Medicine, in its 1998 Position Stand, "The Recommended Quantity and Quality of Exercise for Healthy Adults," says adults should try to stretch every day for health. After you have warmed up and gone for a walk, slow your pace and walk for a few 5-10 more minutes to cool down.

I have to be careful about stretching, however, because the medicine I take for high blood pressure causes foot, calf, and thigh cramps. If I stretch too quickly, I get severe cramps, and they can last for hours. It is best to ease into stretching if you take prescribed medication as I do. Stretching comes with a caution at my age: Stop if you start to hurt. This is good advice for walkers of all ages.

These are just a few examples of stretches. More information about stretching is available from the Internet, specialty magazines and websites.

Resources

1. California Department of Public Health, in cooperation with the Partnership for a Walkable America and the U.S. Department of Transportation, *California Walk Kit,* 2007.

2. Mayo Clinic website, www.mayoclinic.com, "Stretching: Focus on Flexibility."

3. "3 Moves to Stay Strong," *Woman's Day,* February 2013, p. 132.

4. American Heart Association website, www.heart.org, "Stretching and Flexibility Exercises."

5. Mayo Clinic staff, "Happy, Healthy Feet: Exercises for Stability," *Mayo Clinic Health Letter,* February 2013, p.7.

Chapter 5

Getting Out and About

Before you head out, you need to make sure you have comfortable shoes. You have many styles to choose from, too many in my view. Which one will suit you best? Allow plenty of shopping time because finding the right shoes can take a while. I had to go to several stores before I found the kind of shoes I wanted. Over the years women's feet have gotten larger and finding my size, 6 ½ B, wasn't easy.

Bring thick socks, socks that "wick" moisture, with you. Your doctor may have prescribed support hose if you have vein problems. I wear support knee-highs and when I walk, I wear socks over my hose. This way, I have the support and comfort I need. Drug stores carry support socks, but according to my doctor, they don't provide as much support as prescription hose.

Mother Nature doesn't give us identical feet and one of your feet may be slightly larger than the other. Make sure the sales associate measures both of your feet. Try on different styles of shoes and walk around the store a bit. Are both of your feet comfortable? Do you think you could walk a mile or more in these shoes? Other things to think about are listed below.

- Shape of your arch
- Size of the toe box (Your toes shouldn't be touching the end of the shoe.)
- Enough width for swelling feet on a hot day
- Soles that cushion and protect your feet
- Ankle cushion
- Inside pad inserts
- Durability
- Price.

Cost was a major factor for me and it may be for you. I wasn't willing, and still am not willing, to pay $200 or more for walking shoes. At my doctor's suggestion, however, I have purchased orthopedic shoes for everyday and they cost $200. These shoes have worked well and are still comfortable. I try not to walk in shoes that are lacking support, such as espadrilles, but sometimes I've done it, and have always been sorry later.

According to the American Podiatric Medical Association, walking shoes should never be used for running. Replace your shoes after you have walked 300 to 500 miles, earlier if they are uncomfortable. Some health experts recommend new shoes each year because walking regularly flattens the interior cushioning. You may wish to buy two pairs of walking shoes and alternate them.

I bought a pair of walking shoes with cushioned soles, and wore them when I was at the health club. I also bought a pair of European walking shoes, at least, that's what the store owner called them. According to the owner, European women wear this kind of shoe when they go grocery shopping and stroll in the evening after dinner. This was a nice story and I knew it was partially true, for I had seen French women wearing similar shoes, and couples walking arm-in-arm in the evening. Evening walking is common in many European countries and it's a social custom, as well as a health custom.

I liked the lace-up style of shoes because of their ample toe boxes, arch support, and triple cushioning. Since most of my walking is on hard surfaces such as city sidewalks, these are the shoes I wear most often. They were so comfortable I bought a second pair a month later. The important point here is that I tried out the shoes for weeks before I invested in another pair. You could say I "test drove" the shoes, an example you may wish to follow.

I've bought walking shoes from a national discount chain that sells clothing, toys, jewelry, and home goods. When I saw the shoes I was surprised. How the shoes wound up in the store is a mystery. To ensure a proper fit, I tried on both shoes before buying them. For me, comfort is paramount and I know I won't walk if I am not comfortable. As comedian Billy Crystal once said, "I can't be funny if my feet don't feel right."

Your next decision is to whether to wear a pedometer or not.

A pedometer keeps track of your steps. Helpful as it is, using a pedometer is not essential to your fitness program. Instead, you may track your physical activity by measuring distances. If you walk to work, for example, and know the distance from your home to your workplace is a mile, you already have an indication of how far you walk each day. The same is true if you walk to public transportation.

Wearing a pedometer may be a motivator for you. Discount and sports stores carry different types of pedometers and they vary in price. Before you buy a pedometer think about the features you need and the maximum amount you want to spend. Here are some additional things to consider.

- Price may be number one. Do you want to buy a pedometer that will last for a year or will a "cheapie" work just as well?
- When you buy your pedometer, stock up on batteries. I buy batteries in bulk at a big box store.

- Test your pedometer for accuracy. Clip it to your waist, make sure it is set at 0, and walk 20 steps. If your pedometer reads 20 it is accurate.
- Wear your pedometer on the right side. When you clip it to your waist make sure it is centered over your knee and on a straight axis with your leg.
- Measure your stride by taking 10 steps. Then measure this distance with a tape measure. Divide the distance by 10 and that is the length of your stride.
- Wear your pedometer all day.
- Check your pedometer several times a day to make sure it is on straight. A crooked pedometer will miss steps and give you a false reading, which can be discouraging.
- Have an extra pedometer on hand in case your pedometer breaks, falls on the ground, or into the toilet. Yes it happens, and more often than you think. Three women have told me they dropped their pedometers into the toilet, and those are just the ones who admitted it.

The pedometers I've used cost sixteen dollars or less. You might want to buy a high-tech pedometer, a Wireless Activity and Sleep Tracker, for around $99 plus tax. This model is connected to a computer and keeps track of your steps, the distance you have covered, the calories you have burned, and stairs you have climbed. A friend of mine has this type of pedometer and, instead of clipping it to her waist, she tucks it into her bra.

While I admire technology, I think I'll stick with a cheaper pedometer. I don't want to spend that much on a pedometer and I'm not a technical person. Linking the computer and pedometer together would be a challenge for me, such a challenge I would probably give up.

I haven't purchased a new pedometer. Rather than counting steps, I am focusing on 30 minutes of physical activity at least five days a week. So far, I'm doing well, and I can feel the effects of walking in my tummy and thighs. Sometimes I walk at the local mall. Most days, however, I walk in a mega store. Because I walk between eight and nine in the morning, I'm able to avoid crowds and walk at a brisk pace. I walk around the perimeter of the store three-to-four times. Staff members have gotten used to my walking and smile when I go by.

Friends have expressed concern about my mega store walking. "I would keep buying stuff," one admitted. "Do you?"

"No," I answered quickly, "because I know the difference between want and need."

Resources

1. American Podiatric Medical Association website, www.ampa.org, "Preparing Your Feet for a Lifetime of Walking."

2. Mayo Clinic website, www.mayoclinic.com, "Walking Shoes: Features and Fit can Keep You on the Move."

3. Fenton, Mark. *The Complete Guide to Walking for Health, Weight Loss and Fitness. Guilford,* CT, 2001.

4. American College of Sports Medicine website, www.acsm.org, "ACSM Fit Society Page," Spring 2005, "Walkee Talkee: Answers to Pedometer Questions."

5. Fenton, Mark. *The Complete Guide to Walking for Health, Weight Loss and Fitness.* Guilford, CT: *Walking Magazine,* 2001.

Chapter 6

Healthy Snacks for You

Starting out with a good breakfast is like filling your car with gas; you have fuel for the day. Your breakfast could include juice, plain strawberries, whole grain cereal or whole grain bread, and low-fat or skim milk. Eating two fruits for breakfast will help you reach a nutrition goal of five fruits and vegetables, or more, per day. Be aware of your serving sizes, and don't overeat before walking.

According to a Mayo Clinic website article, eating too much before physical activity can make you sluggish. You don't want to start your walk feeling like a sloth. Besides, you won't enjoy your walk it your tummy is too full.

Pack a healthy snack if you think you will get hungry. Read the nutrition information on all products before you buy them. Some so-called health bars, for example, are really sweet cookies in disguise. Choose low sugar, sugar-free, low-salt, or salt-free foods. Nature's self-packaged fruits, apples, bananas, and pears, are healthy snacks for walking.

Doctors know consuming too much salt makes the heart work harder. I'm a salt-sensitive person and so is my husband. After he received his new aorta, I was extra careful about the meals I prepared. Bread, the staff of life in America, can contain lots of salt. I bought a bread machine and made all of our own bread. Recipes were included with the bread maker and I made many of them, but with less salt.

Though I occasionally use mixes, I try to avoid them because of the high salt and ingredients I can barely pronounce. Now I was extra careful and spent hours on meal preparation. Soup was a problem because good soup needs salt. I substituted herbs for the salt and my soup was pretty good. "I couldn't do what you're doing," my sister-in-law commented.

"You do what you have to do," I replied.

To eat healthy you need to become a food label detective. I read every word on every label and pay special attention to salt, fat, and sugar. Too much sugar can contribute to weight gain and obesity. In 2009 the American Heart Association noted a relationship between excess sugar and metabolic abnormalities, and recommended cutting back on sugars, advising women to consume "no more than 100 [sugar] calories a day, or about six teaspoons."

This isn't very much sugar and you may be eating more than you realize.

Sugar has many names: high fructose corn syrup, molasses, maple syrup, cane sugar, glucose, maltose, sucrose, and honey. Each gram of sugar contains four calories. If the nutrition label says the product 15 grams of sugar per serving, you are getting 60 calories from sugar *alone*. One of the quickest ways to lose weight, according to Mayo Clinic, is to cut back on sugar, and I did that.

I could see the results, a thinner me, in three weeks. Thankfully, I'm not a dessert person, and it doesn't take much willpower to say "no" to gooey cake. Still, I'm always on the lookout for hidden sugar. For example, I use fat-free half and half in my coffee.

Corn syrup solids are the second ingredient on the list, adding two grams of sugar per two tablespoons of cream. Though I still use this product, I factor this sugar into my daily intake.

Ketchup is a source of hidden sugar, or as a relative declared, "Ketchup is a sugar delivery system." Read the label and sugar is probably the second ingredient. This doesn't mean you have to give up ketchup forever. Buy the brand with the lowest sugar content. Instead of eating unlimited ketchup, limit yourself to one tablesoon. Most nutrition experts have veered away from the idea of forbidden foods, and say we can eat all foods in moderate amounts.

You're probably asking yourself, "Can I eat fast food?" Yes, if you order carefully. During our travels my husband and I have eaten fast food and we've been amazed at the service we received. When we asked for French fries without salt, a staff person cooked them especially for us. Skim or reduced fat milk was always available and there were many salad options. Some fast food restaurants also have mixed fruit. When it comes to hamburgers, a plain one, without cheese or bacon, is the healthiest choice.

When I'm hungry I often eat a small dish of unsweetened applesauce. I also like pears and prefer to eat them when they are crunchy. Plain walnuts and unsalted peanuts are also some of my snack foods. Sometimes I eat plain, reduced salt popcorn. What are some healthy snacks you could eat while walking?

- A banana. Though it's high in calories (200) and carbohydrate (51 grams) one banana also contains 806 milligrams of potassium, which can counteract leg cramps.
- Raw carrot sticks or baby carrots. These are easy to pack, keep well, are low in calories, contain Vitamins A, C, K and others. They also contain calcium.
- Peanut butter on whole grain crackers. A couple of cracker sandwiches in your pocket may be just the boost you need.

- Energy granola bar. This recommendation comes from the University of Tennessee Medical Center. "Kashi brand works well," the center notes.
- Dried fruit. You need to be careful here because dried fruit is loaded with sugar. Look for the fruit with the lowest sugar content.
- A small handful of breakfast cereal, such as Cheerios.
- A fresh apple. Wash the apple first. You may also slice it and squeeze lemon juice on the slices to prevent them from turning brown.
- Nuts. These are a smart choice because many nuts are rich in omega-3 fatty acids, the ones that help your heart. Some medical experts think nuts can reduce the risk of blood clots and heart attack. Nuts also contain fiber and Vitamin E. Choose unsalted nuts.
- Melba toast crackers. Pick the ones with the most whole grain, such as rye and pumpernickel.
- Low-fat cheese. When it comes to cheese, fat content and size matter. Your snack should only be as large as two dominoes.
- Fat-free popcorn. Pop the corn and spoon ¼ cup servings into plastic snack bags.
- Homemade trail mix. Since commercial trail mix can be pricey, you may want to make your own. Mix equal parts breakfast cereal (such as crisp, round oats) with chocolate chips, chopped walnuts, and chopped dried apricots. Or mix fat-free popcorn with almonds and raisins. Experiment until you find the combinations you like. Spoon ¼-cup servings into plastic snack bags.

Because it is cheaper than commercial products, and I can control the ingredients, I make my own granola. My basic recipe comes from *The Healthy Cook*, published by *Prevention* magazine. It calls for wheat germ, something I'm not too fond of, so I deleted it from the recipe. If you like wheat germ, substitute one cup of wheat germ for one cup of oatmeal. Store the granola in an airtight container.

Granola with Walnuts and Apples

Ingredients:

6 cups quick cooking oatmeal

1 teaspoon ground cinnamon

¼ cup honey

2 tablespoons extra light olive oil

2 tablespoons apple or orange juice

1 teaspoon pure vanilla extract

½ cup walnut pieces or sliced almonds

1 cup dried apples, chopped and added later

Method:

Preheat your oven to 300 degrees. Coat two rimmed baking pans with non-stick spray. In a large bowl, combine oatmeal and cinnamon. In a glass measuring cup combine honey, olive oil, juice, and vanilla extract. Microwave mixture on a high setting for one minute. Stir, add to oatmeal, and toss well. Spoon granola onto baking sheets, spreading it out evenly. Bake for 20 minutes, stirring several times, until granola starts to brown. Transfer granola to a large bowl and add dried apples. This recipe makes about seven cups. You may omit the nuts and add an extra half cup of chopped dried apples if you wish.

Good plain, this granola also tastes good with low-fat yogurt and sprinkled on top of fresh fruit. Are you stumped on a gift? Homemade granola in an attractive jar, tied with a bow, makes a great gift for a relative or friend.

Resources

1. American Heart Association website, www.heart.org, "Association Recommends Reduced Intake of Added Sugars."

2. American Heart Association website, www.heart.org, "Sugars and Carbohydrates."

3. Mayo Clinic website, www.mayoclinic.com, "Eating and Exercise: 5 tips to Maximize Your Workouts."

4. University of Tennessee Medical Center website, www.utmedicalcenter.org, "Walking, Running, Hiking: Fall Activity Essential Snacks."

5. Hoffman, Matthew and Joachim, David, Editors. *The Healthy Cook*. Emmaus, PA, 1997, p. 177.

Chapter 7

Safety is Always First

You have to make your own safety plan and it depends on how far you are going to walk. A major hike requires special planning. Other circumstances, such as city construction projects and road work, should factor into your plan. If you are an epileptic, or have other physical challenges, wear a medic alert bracelet. I carry a list of the medications I take in my wallet. Please follow these safety tips, starting with hydration.

Staying hydrated is one of the best things you can do for yourself. Drink water before you walk and bring water with you. Older people like me sometimes mistake thirst for hunger. Before I have a snack, I ask myself, "Am I really hungry or am I thirsty?" Most often, I'm thirsty, and I'm glad I know because it stops me from eating too much.

Always plan ahead. If you're going on a long hike bring a healthy snack with you, food that's easy to carry, such as trail mix, nuts, or an apple. Since I usually walk after breakfast or lunch so I don't need a snack. I avoid walking with a full stomach, however, because it makes me uncomfortable. It also slows me down.

Walking with a friend or group is another way to stay safe. One walking buddy can keep you on the fitness path and three or four are even better. Women can encourage each other, and as time passes, you and your friends meld into a walking team. And team spirit is contagious. All I can say is, "You go girls!"

Use community crosswalks. In Minnesota, this is easy in the spring, summer, and fall, but it can be a challenge in the winter, when the crosswalks are covered with snow. Corner snow piles also get progressively higher, freeze in place, and obscure traffic. I peek around the snow piles before I step forward. Wherever you live, take advantage of the crosswalks because they exist to keep you safe.

Observe traffic signals. Cross on green only and never take chances with yellow. I'm originally from New York State and when I took driver's education in high school, I was trained to yield on yellow. All too often, at least in my city, drivers accelerate and race through yellow lights, a dangerous practice with oncoming traffic. I don't want to be in the way of a speeding driver and you don't either. Be on the lookout for drivers who aren't looking out for you.

Always have identification on you. Tie your ID to a shoelace, put it in your backpack or fanny pack, or wear it on a lanyard. Years ago, a Minnesota runner was severely injured on a country road. I don't recall the circumstances of her injury, but I do know she didn't carry any identification, and it took hours for the police to identify the woman and contact her family. I belong to the Minnesota Medical Association Alliance, an affiliate of Minnesota Medical Association, and this story led to a health project, shoelace identification tags. Whether it's on your shoelace, in your pocket, or attached to a lanyard, make sure you have ID with you.

Wear reflective clothing at dusk and at night. Reflective clothing is available from discount and sports stores. Or you can save money by putting reflective tape on regular clothing. Wearing white clothing also helps drivers to see you. One evening, when I was driving, I had to swerve suddenly to avoid hitting a runner totally dressed in black. He was wearing black running pants, a black jacket, and a black hat. But he wasn't wearing reflective clothing, anything white that would reflect light, or a head lamp. Please don't make this mistake!

Toss your cellphone in a fanny pack or back pack. Make sure your phone is fully charged before you head out. You know this, yet may forget to charge your phone.

Bring an extra shoelace. If you've ever broken a shoelace while you're out and about, you know it's a bummer. One shoe feels fine and the other feels like it's going to fall off at any minute. I've had to tie knots in shoelaces while traveling. Now, before I leave the house, I always check my shoelaces.

Protecting your face with a cap or hat is one of the best safety measures you can take. The cap should have a visor that shields your entire face, not just your forehead and eyes. Usually I wear a cap, but in the summer I wear a wide-brimmed straw hat. It's one of those hats you can roll up, put in a suitcase, take it out, unroll it, and it still retains its shape. I think of it as my "trick" hat. Depite all the rolling, the hat is still in good condition.

Protect your skin with sunscreen. Your skin can be damaged by the sun in cloudy weather, not just sunny. Choose sunscreen that has a SPF 15 rating or higher. Be sure to apply it to the back of your neck and under your chin. Since I take a prescribed antibiotic each day, I'm supposed to stay out of the sun. My husband bought me a sunblock product that has a protection rating of 70. It's oil-free, fragrance-free, and shields six layers of skin, according to the label. Your pharmacy should be able to provide more information about sunscreen brands.

Use insect repellant. Locals joke about the mosquito being the state bird, but insect bites, especially itchy, red mosquito welts, can make you miserable. Mosquitoes can be dangerous and have caused West Nile Virus, Encephalitis, Dengue, Yellow Fever, St. Louis Encephalitis, Malaria and other disease in the US, according to the American Mosquito Control Association. I use insect repellant if I walk in the woods or at night. Apply the repellant carefully because it dissolves nail polish and damages plastic eyeglass lenses.

Putting tissues in your pocket isn't a safety tip, it's really a comfort tip. Cold weather can cause your nose to run and it's nice to have tissues handy. Both my husband and I take medications that make our noses run, so tissues are a must for us.

If you're far from home or close, it's wise to bring a travel poncho. We were caught in a downpour so intense the rain penetrated our raincoats. My skirt felt like it had just come out of the washing machine, and my husband's slacks were so wet he smelled like a wet wool blanket. Thankfully, we were able to find plastic ponchos at a drug store for six dollars each. Though we looked like we were wearing plastic table cloths, we didn't care because we were dry.

Vary your walking schedule. Predators look for patterns they can use to their advantage. I'm sorry to say there are predators out there and, to confuse them, vary your walking time and route.

Reporting unsafe conditions helps to keep all walkers safe. This tip comes from the International Walk to School Day program and its "Walkability Checklist." The first question on the list: Did you have room to walk? The list asks you to watch for cracked sidewalks, uneven sidewalks, no sidewalks, blown street light bulbs, downed tree branches, obstructed stop signs, unsafe crosswalks, and congested areas that need "traffic calming." If you see any of these things report them to the appropriate government agency or department.

Be observant. Recently my husband and I volunteered at the public library. When we left it was raining so hard there was standing water in the streets. During the night this water froze and turned streets and sidewalks into ice rinks. In the morning I opened the garage door to check the driveway and saw large, frozen footprints. The footprints came down the hill, went to the garage service door, seemed to turn around and cross in front of the garage doors, and continued across the lawn. The footprints were too large to be my husband's footprints.

Why did the person go to the side door? I remembered a robbery that had occurred a block away. The family had forgotten to lock the garage service door and back door of their house. While they slept, robbers came into the house and stole several television sets and any small electrics they could find. The person who made the footprints could have been checking to see if our service door was locked. Much as I love to walk in the neighborhood, now my neighborhood doesn't seem as safe.

Still, we need to keep walking for heart health. Remember, the American Heart Association recommends *30 minutes of physical activity per day*. There is safety in numbers, and that's why it's wise to have a walking buddy or buddies.

Bring medications with you. My husband carries extra medications in his pocket as a safety precaution. I'm on an aspirin regimen prescribed by my physician to prevent heart attack and stroke. Though I take a low-dose aspirin (between 81 and 325 milligrams) each morning, I carry extra aspirin in my purse in case I have a heart attack. You may wish to do the same.

Call 911 immediately if you start to have the symptoms of heart attack. The 911 operator may, or may not, ask you to take an aspirin. According to the American Heart Association (AHA), research findings show taking an aspirin can improve your chances of surviving a heart attack. In a Family Health Guide website article, Harvard Medical School recommends *chewing* one adult aspirin, not swallowing it whole.

"For the best results, chew a single full-sized 325-mg tablet," the article advises. This should be a plain aspirin, not one that is coated. You should not take an aspirin if you think you're having a stroke, however. For me, having aspirin within reach is more than a safety precaution; it is comforting. When I went to buy aspirin at the local drug store, I couldn't find any uncoated tablets and asked the pharmacist for help. He found the brand that was least coated.

"This will still help," he explained. "It will taste like crap, but the coating will be gone in seconds."

"Crap is okay if you're having a heart attack," I retorted. As soon as I returned home, I tucked the new bottle of aspirin in my purse.

Resources

1. U.S. Department of Transportation, Partnership for a Walkable America, "Walkability Checklist."
2. Mayo Clinic website, www.MayoClinic.com, "Walking Safety: Avoid Potential Pitfalls."
3. American Heart Association website, www.heart.org, "Aspirin and Heart
4. Disease."
5. Harvard Medical School website, www.hms.harvard.edu, Family Health Guide, "Aspirin for Heart Attack: Chew or Swallow?"
6. American Mosquito Control Association website, www.mosquito.org, "Mosquito- Bourne Diseases."

Chapter 8

Staying on the Fitness Path

Life can change the best of plans. Before you know it, you have taken a detour, and are far off the fitness path. While this can be upsetting, these tips can get you back on track. You don't have to follow all the tips at once. Pick one or two and start working on them. Check off each tip as you complete it. Even if you follow only one tip, you have been proactive about your health.

- **Eat healthy foods and normal servings**. Do you know the difference between a portion and a serving? Many people don't, and you may be one of them. A portion is the amount of food you choose to eat, such as the food you pile on your plate at an all-you-can-eat buffet. A serving is a measured amount of food based on nutrition data. Try to eat normal servings and consume fruits and vegetables first to quell your hunger.

- **Put walking on your calendar**. Think of walking as an appointment you must keep. This tip comes from Mayo Clinic and I can assure you, it works. Seeing your walking "appointments" in writing makes them look important, and you don't want to miss one. Draw a star next to these walking appointments to imprint them in your mind. Keep telling yourself, "I'm walking for me."

- **Continue to set goals.** After I lost five pounds my next goal was to lose five more. I've worked towards my goals slowly and, according to nutrition experts, this is the way to do it. Do you have a friend who is living successfully with heart disease? If so, you may wish to talk with her. What are her goals? Do you have any goals in common?

- **Divide big goals into smaller parts.** small goals makes it easier to reach a large goal. Tracking your progress is also easier. I was really inspired when the waistband on my slacks was an inch and a half too big, a fact that proved my walking and eating programs were working. My initial weight loss nudged me forward to my main goal, reaching the size that used to be normal for me, size eight.

- **Check your shoes.** Over time, walking shoes show interior and exterior wear. Replace your shoes if necessary. Watch for summer and after-Christmas sales because you can really find some bargains. I haven't had good luck with mail order shoes, however. The fit seems to depend on where the shoes were made. Sending them back is a hassle and you have to pay the return postage.

- **Check your socks.** I tried wearing regular, patterned socks from a discount store and they had holes in them by the second wearing. Plain socks, and ones made specifically for walking, are best. Discard any socks that have holes. I'm a thirifty person and, though I've tried mending socks, it hasn't worked, and the bumps make me feel like I have pebbles in my shoes.

- **Vary your walking buddies**. Ask a good friend to come with you or a new neighbor you have just met. I'm sure she will appreciate the invitation. Who knows, in addition to being a walking friend, she may become a best friend. Your walking sisters are a marvelous group and you may as well take advantage of them.

- **Start a walking group.** Be sure to use the Walking Buddies page in this guide. Keep the group going by varying your route, walking type, and your rewards. Your walking buddies may become a support group, something that is good to have at any age and stage of life.

- **Bring kids along.** Your fitness model has an impact on children's lives and grandchildren's lives. Invite children to come with you. I guarantee, you'll have more fun on your walks. Seeing the world through a children's eyes helps me to re-discover the world, and that is a blessing.

- **Cut yourself some slack.** Fitness is a goal that takes time to reach and is worth your time. I have to be careful not to sabotage myself. One day I was so pleased with my weight loss I rewarded myself with food, a foolish mistake. I was ashamed of myself and couldn't believe I had done that. Thank goodness I was able to come up with the self-talk I needed.

- **Always have an alternate plan.** Be prepared for weather changes, school closings, and illness. When my husband came down with the flu, my daily schedule and meal preparation changed. One of the first things I did was make chicken soup for him. I walked alone that day.

- **Walk in place.** Get in a few extra steps while you're waiting for coffee to brew, talking on the phone, or watching television. You will be amazed at the number of steps you accrue.

Are you on hold or caught in one of those telephone loops that go from extension one, to extension two, and continue on until you're back where you started? Walk in place to make the waiting easier and dilute your anger.

- **Turn walking into an event.** Go for a bird walk, historic walk, or nature walk. As spring draws closer, I look for buds on trees and tiny green shoots in gardens. The arrival of spring is an event in Minnesota and everyone celebrates it. Like soldiers emerging from bunkers, people come out of their homes, walk around their houses or apartments, and stare in amazement at greening shrubs and budding flowers. All of my friends watch for the first robin, proof that spring has come again.

- **Vary your time and route.** This is a good safety measure and makes your walks more interesting. For example, walking early in the morning feels different from walking at dusk. I love early morning and have found, in all my years of living, that it's my most productive time of day. By dusk, I'm starting to wind down, yawning a bit, and thinking of bed.

- **Participate in charity walks.** I've only participated in one fundraising walk and it was on a health club track. The event raised funds to provide clean water for an African village. Walking with friends was fun and we felt like we were making a difference.

- **Keep rewarding yourself**. You started out on the fitness path and are still on it!

If you belong to a walking group, members may wish to have a celebration of some kind, a special walk, a field trip, a heart healthy dinner. You could even exchange heart healthy recipes.

Maybe you're reading this book because you were diagnosed with heart disease or at risk for it. WomenHeart, a national coalition for women with the disease, may be beneficial to you. The organization has published a "Heart Health Action Kit." To order a kit go to www.womenheart.org, and complete the ordering information. Don't make the mistake I made and forget to submit your information. As soon as your request is received, WomenHeart will send you an email with your username and password.

As a health and wellness writer, I've accumulated a small library of resources. recent acquisitions include resources about making healthy restaurant choices, heart function, and heart-healthy cooking. Best of all, I've learned how to modify recipes automatically. I substitute unsweetened applesauce for shortening, use a low-calorie sugar blend for baking, cook with fat-free milk and olive oil, and substitute herbs for salt.

By the way, though the salt shaker was banished from our table years ago, I continue to be a food label detective. Some brands of lemon pepper, a product I like and use, have hidden salt in them. If a product claims to be pepper, why does it contain salt? This doesn't seem right to me. I've learned that a product that lists salt as the first ingredient contains more salt than I want.

Because I'm allergic to soy, I must read every word on every food label, and this slows my shopping. Soy has many names: soy protein, soy meal, soy flour, tofu, and other product names. All cause me intense abdominal pain. So many people are allergic to soy that many manufacturers now include it in their ingredients lists. In addition to looking for soy, I pay attention to the sugar content. Since manufacturers "fudge" on the serving size to make products look healthier, I check the serving size. Recently I've come across products that list half a serving as the normal size. Nobody I know eats only a half cup of mac and cheese, that's for sure.

To stay on a fitness path we must be savvy shoppers!

Chapter 9

Proactive Steps to Take

It's true. Genetics and illness play a part in heart health. Both my husband and I have heart-related issues and both of us have become more proactive about our health. Every day, we try to take good care of ourselves and our hearts. Scarlet Fever is rare today, thanks to the invention of antibiotics, but that doesn't alter my medical history. Indeed, Scarlet Fever changed my life forever.

I caught the disease when I was eight or nine years old, and remember being sick because I was *so* sick. Our family doctor came to the house and checked me over. He treated me like an adult and that's why I liked him. Antibiotics were not available at the time, and the only thing my parents and I could do was wait, watch, and hope. Someone from public health came to our house and stuck a large QUARANTINED sign at the curb. The sign really upset our neighbors and they stayed far away from us. While they would call "Hello!" from across the street, they wouldn't come any closer.

A milk truck delivered dairy products to our neighborhood. Usually the milkman usually left our order of two gallons in a small, insulated box by the back door. After the quarantine sign went up he left milk at the curb and sped away. "Look where he left the milk!" my mother exclaimed. Annoying as this was, things became worse, because the bread truck also stopped coming. This made me sad because my mother, who was an excellent baker, often bought cupcakes from the truck. I can still see them in my mind, six cupcakes in a cardboard box, two with vanilla frosting, two with chocolate, and two with strawberry, my favorite flavor. Between the fleeing milkman, no bread truck, and frightened neighbors, my parents felt very isolated.

From my upstairs bedroom I could hear them lamenting about the sign. As soon as I felt better, I got out of bed, went downstairs, and peered out the porch windows to see if the sign was really there. It was and it was big. When I share my quarantine story with others they look at me in surprise. Though isolating people and products because of disease is less common today, the Centers for Disease Control and Prevention (CDC) still maintains quarantine centers in strategic cities.

Scarlet Fever damaged my heart valve, but it wasn't something I thought about or worried about very much. Today, the "woo-sha" sound is louder and more pronounced, and I'm walking to help my heart. If you are at risk for heart disease or living with a damaged heart, you can take action for heart health. These aren't complex steps, they are easy steps, and each one is worth the effort. Indeed, they may prolong your life.

New genetics research may also prolong your life. Today, medical treatment is individualized, based on your genetic history and medical history. Still, there are older adults like me who have heart murmurs and faulty aortas. My husband's story is more dramatic than my Scarlet Fever story.

In 1997 the lining of his aorta severed on the way to work. "I could feel it go down from my chest and to my thigh," he recalled.

"The pain was intense." A Mayo Clinic physician specializing in internal medicine and aerospace medicine, he knew he was in trouble, and headed for the nearest Trauma Center. At the time, the center was doing some construction work near the entrance, and my husband couldn't get the car as close as he wanted. Fortunately, a workman spotted him and rushed to his aid. My husband knew many staff members, including the chief of the Trauma Center, because he had been the head of employee health for years.

"What's your diagnosis?" the chief asked.

"I think my aorta dissected," my husband replied. It turned out his diagnosis was correct. During his week-long hospitalization my elder daughter, who was alive then, brought the twins to see him. They were quiet and somber when saw grandpa hooked up to so many wires and machines.

"What's wrong with him?" they asked.

"He has a broken heart," our daughter replied, attempting to explain a complex medical condition to her young children.

Months later my grandson, a "techie" from birth, told my husband, "You had two television sets over your bed. One had numbers on it and the other had lines." Of course, they weren't tevision sets, they were medical monitors. Today, when I think about my grandson's observation, I smile. He is a college junior now, in an honors program, on the Dean's List, and headed for MD and PhD degrees.

The twins drew pictures for their grandpa and the nursing staff hung them on the wall across from his bed. There were four pictures and one was a drawing of a large, in-tact Valentine heart, not a broken one. I think it was drawn by my granddaughter. The heart drawing may have been her way of healing her sick grandpa.

My husband's primary physician measured the size of his aorta regularly. Despite these measures and many prescription medications, the lining of his aorta continued to expand, and he had to have surgery. When my husband was wheeled into surgery I started to cry and he did, too. Would this be the last time I saw him? The invasive surgery took hours and I was worried sick the whole time.

Thankfully, the surgery was successful and my husband was transferred to intensive care. A technician came to his bedside to take an x-ray of his chest. "Take a deep breath," the technician said. My husband took a deep breath and his chest went such spasms he was incapable of taking another breath. The technician called to his nurse, who was across the room. His male nurse, whom he later described as being "built like a football linebacker," managed to get him breathing again.

"I must have blacked out for a few seconds," my husband recalled, "because the next thing I remember is the nurse pounding on my chest." Thank goodness his nurse was just a few steps away.

We belonged to the hospital's health club and had been exercising there for months. Every time I visited my husband, I went to the club and walked on a treadmill. I shared my anxieties with one of the staff members. She was sympathetic and commented, "I like it when people exercise to reduce stress." Walking helped me during this time and I think it will help you manage the stressful times in your life.

Years have passed since my husband's surgery and it has given him a second chance at life. Every time I see the large durved scar that starts on my husband's chest, goes around the side of his body, and ends in the middle of his back, I want to cry for all he went through. I also want to cheer for modern medicine and the healthcare team that took such good care of him. Today, we are walking advocates and think of walking as a proactive step.

Here are some proactive steps you may take for heart health. The first one may be the most important.

- Get a check-up each year, including blood pressure, cholesterol, and diabetes screening.
- Know your blood pressure.
- Know your HDL (good cholesterol) and LDL (bad cholesterol) levels. Your HDL should be 60 mg/dL or more.
- Know your BMI – body mass index.
- Maintain a healthy weight.
- Get at least seven hours of sleep a night.
- Eat 5-10 servings of fruits and vegetables a day and a low-fat diet.
- Twice a week, eat fish that contains Omega-3 oils (salmon, mackerel, herring, sardines, fresh tuna.)
- Or, take 1,000 mg. of fish oil a day. It has to be the right kind of fish oil, however, so check with your doctor.
- Floss your teeth regularly.
- Don't smoke. If you do smoke, join a smoking cessation program.
- Get 30 minutes of physical activity a day, most days of the week.
- Stand more often. When you travel and are in a motel, set your computer on the ironing board and stand as you work. You may also walk around the perimeter of your hotel room. I attended a two-day conference in Minneapolis. When I was in my room, I turned on the television and walked 1,000 steps around my room each day.
- Know the symptoms of heart attack. Men's symptoms include shortness of breath, feeling weak, unusual fatigue, cold sweats, dizziness. Women's symptoms include disturbed sleep, unusual fatigue, shortness of breath, in some,

upper back pressure, indigestion, anxiety. You may think you have the flu.

- If you are at risk of heart attack, take one low-dose aspirin per day. Check with your doctor first, however.
- Control stress with yoga, meditation, or walking meditation.

I've been amazed at the stress-reducing power of walking. Something happens to your thinking when you are moving and, though you have the same problems at the end of a walk, they seem less threatening. Your mood shifts and solutions may start to emerge. If you're on stress overload now, take a walk instead of taking a nap. Walk regularly and you will be amazed at the results. Think of your heart sisters while you are walking.

Resources

1. American Heart Association website, www.heart.org, "Heart Attack Symptoms in Women."
2. Mann, Denise. "Heart Attacks in Women: Different Symptoms, Different Outcomes," WebMD website, www.webmd.com.
3. Mayo Clinic website, www.mayoclinic.com, "5 Medication-Free Strategies to Help Prevent Heart Disease."
4. Mayo Clinic website, www.mayoclinic.com, "Heart Attack Symptoms: Know What's a Medical Emergency."
5. US Department of Health and Human Services website, www.womenshealth.gov "Heart Disease."

Chapter 10

Walking after Heart Surgery

After heart surgery your doctor will prescribe an aftercare program to support and speed recovery. Aftercare has many aspects: pain management, incision care, bathing instructions, diet, physical activity, emotional health, and sexuality. Your aftercare program depends on the type of surgery, medication adjustment (if necessary), how well your incision is healing, and whether or not your lungs are clear.

In my husband's case, his lungs were clear, but his pleura, a membrane that envelops the lung, was filled with fluid. This frustrated both of us. He had come through surgery well, was eager to go home, and I was eager for him to be home. We ignored our frustrations and focused on what needed to be done. A drainage tube was inserted in my husband's chest and he was fed intravenously for 10 days.

"I was never hungry," he later commented.

Several times, I walked with him around the nursing station and I could tell when he was feeling better. I could also tell when he was in acute pain. Finally, he was released from the hospital. He recovered on the living room couch, propped up with pillows and snuggled under a blanket. While this wasn't an ideal arrangement, it made him feel connected to the daily routine and to me.

WebMD offers some aftercare recommendations in its article, "Helping a Loved One Recover from Heart Surgery." Gradually increasing your physical activity is one recommendation. You need to pace yourself, take care of yourself, and, with your doctor's permission, walk every day. "Your doctor or cardiac rehabilitation specialist will give you guidelines for walking," the article explains.

I remember the day my husband went for his initial walk in the neighborhood. We started out slowly and I felt like I was walking in slow motion. The first block had a gradual incline, a good thing for someone recovering from corrective surgery. We had only walked halfway, however, when my husband began to tire, so we turned around and went home. Our expectations fizzled in seconds.

Days passed, and my husband gradually increased his walking distance. The day he walked three blocks was a day of celebration. I wanted to give him a balloon bouquet, launch fireworks in recognition of his achievement, and cue in a cheering crowd. Actually, he did get a cheer. One of our neighbors, who must have heard about my husband's surgery, drove by and called, "Hi John. Good for you!"

Walking can help you recover from surgery. According to the "Mayo Clinic Health Letter," it is common for cardiologists to recommend regular physical activity. "A heart condition may limit a few people, but once it's adequately treated, most heart doctors advise a graduated exercise program," the newsletter notes.

For years, my friend Barbara suffered from irregular heartbeats, (arrhythmias) and they kept getting worse. Her cardiologist recommended a procedure called ablation. A catheter, a long, flexible tube, was inserted into a vein in her thigh, and slowly advanced until it reached her heart. The surgeon identified the area of the heart that was causing the irregular heartbeats, and zapped it with a radio frequency to destroy the tissues.

"It fixed the problem," Barbara declared. "People who have ablation can live normal lives. My surgeon told me he treated a professional football player (he didn't tell me his name) with ablation and he plays in every game."

Recovering from this procedure takes several months. To aid her recovery, Barbara's cardiologist recommended a walking program. "Start slowly," he said, "and keep walking even if it is just two minutes a day. Increase it to three minutes and then four." Barbara bought a treadmill and followed her doctor's advice. But when she started walking on the treadmill she noticed some extra heartbeats. Worried and frightened, Barbara called her doctor.

"Stop, catch your breath, and get back on the treadmill," he advised. Barbara's health improved, continues to improve, and she has become a walking advocate.

This may be a good time to start an aftercare walking log, noting the date, how far you walked, how long you walked, and how you felt while walking. For example, if you get short of breath like my husband, this is something to note. Dizziness and weakness in the legs are other things to note in your log. When you make your entries, be as specific as possible because this information helps your doctor to help you.

Today, many hospitals have support groups for recovering cardiac patients. Members share their personal stories and feelings in group meetings. Sharing helps them identify their feelings, name them, process them, and connect with people who understand their experience. One organization, WomenHeart, runs support groups *specifically* for women living with heart disease.

WomenHeart also has a "Sister Match" program that provides phone and online support. According to coalition surveys, these support services enhance the quality of members' lives, help them follow prescribed treatments and therapies, and improve personal communication. In other words, these women know support is available and that they are not alone. Go to the WomenHeart website for more information about support networks.

Resources

1. Mayo Clinic, *Heart Surgery and You: A Guide for Teens*, Rochester, MN: Mayo Press, 1996, p. 18.

2. WebMD website, www.webmd.com, ""Helping a Loved One Recover From Heart Surgery."

3. Cleveland Clinic website, www.myclevelandclinic.org, "Heart Surgery Recovery,"

4. Emails from Carol Allred, WomenHeart National Coalition for Women With Heart Disease.

5. Phone interview with recovering heart surgery patient

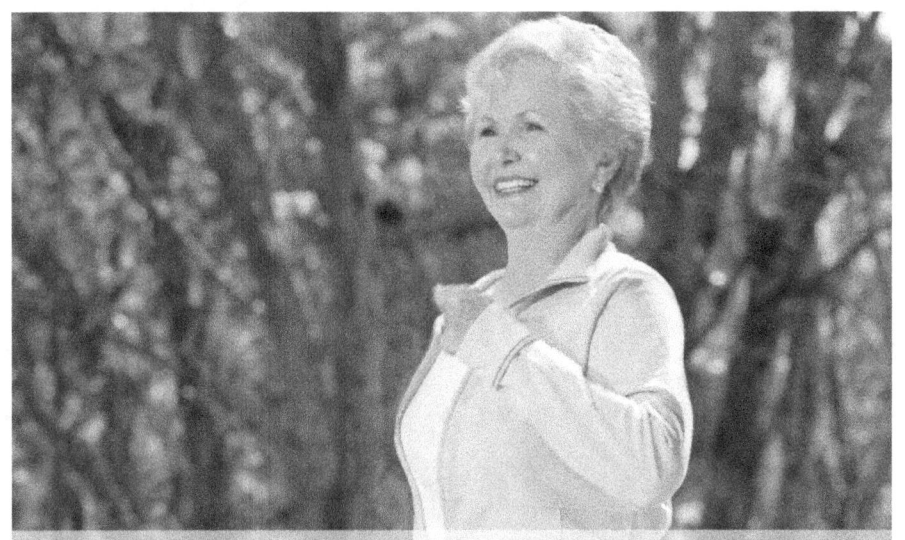

TRACKING AND QUOTES:
YOUR FITNESS MOTIVATION

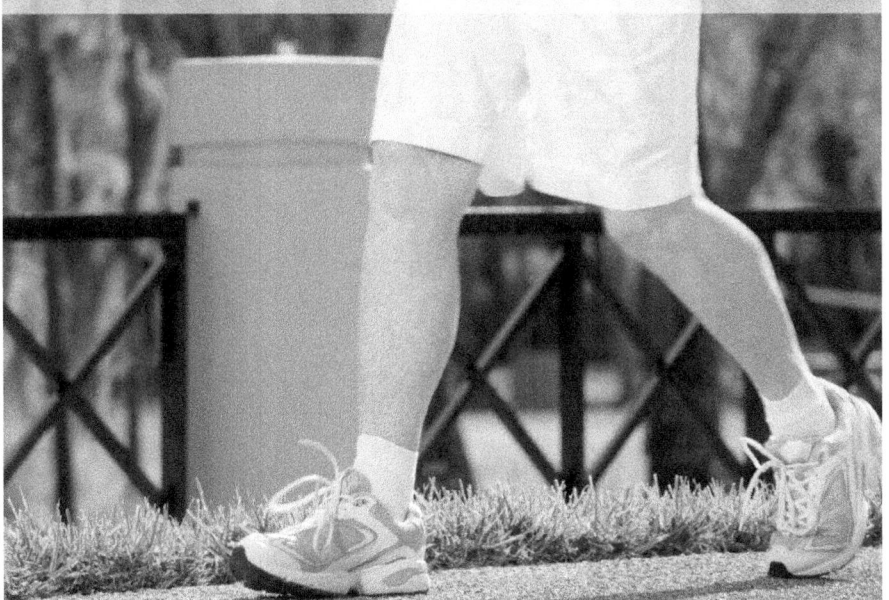

Walking Buddies

This section focuses on three types of motivation, walking buddies, keeping a log, and memorable words. Each motivation type has specific benefits. Finding some walking buddies keeps you in touch with friends who enjoy walking and also provides companionship. You may also meet new friends, swap stories, and laugh together. In case you're wondering, your dog counts as a walking buddy.

Use the buddies page to organize a walking group in your area. You don't need many people, just three will do. Once you're organized, share this list with other members and ask each one to recruit a buddy. It's nice to get a few more members because there will be times when a buddy is ill or traveling or working on a family problem. Walking buddies can be the difference between physical activity and no activity.

Barbara, the person you read about earlier, relied on her walking buddies for motivation until she moved to a small town in Northern Minnesota. She hardly knew anybody in her new community, and lack of companionship had an impact on her fitness program. She asked herself, "If my buddies aren't waiting for me, do I really want to go?" Though Barbara still walks, she walks alone on her treadmill, and it isn't the same as before.

"I miss my buddies a lot," she admitted. "Buddies make a difference."

One buddy can keep you on a healthy path. Are you looking for some walking buddies? Create a walking kit for a friend, with a copy of this book, a water bottle, a pedometer, and some healthy snacks. Invite her to join your group. Your friend will appreciate this gift and it could even change her life. You may also give this gift to a newcomer in your community.

Stay in touch with your walking buddies. Send them email reminders, such as "I'm looking forward to our walk today." Or, "It's raining. Do you want to walk at the mall?" To make you feel like a team, the members of your walking group may wish to wear the same color t-shirts or sweatshirts. Custom-made t-shirts are reasonably priced today. You could design a t-shirt for your group and have them made locally.

Walking Buddies Form

Name   **Phone # or Email**

_____

_____

_____

_____

_____

_____

_____

_____

_____

_____

_____

_____

_____

_____

_____

_____

_____

_____

_____

_____

_____

Keeping a Log

The following pages show you the basic log format and get you started with tracking. Some commercial logs ask you to enter your heart rate and other information. While this is helpful, a simple log is also helpful. Start your log on these pages and continue it in a spiral bound notebook, three-ring binder, or blank journal. A calendar may also be used as a log. Before you buy a calendar, make sure it has large enough squares for entries.

Walking log software is available from the Internet. To learn more about it go to www.walk-log.com. The Webwalking USA website has a free walking map you may access and print out. A friend of mine is tracking her walking distances on a similar map. Her trek began in California and she has been adding steps ever since. "I'm halfway across America!" she exclaimed with a smile. Pedometer logs are something else you may wish to try.

Every once in a while, look through your log, and recall some of your best walks. What made them special? Are there any you want to repeat? Which ones made you smile? Did you learn anything while you were walking?

Walking Woman

Sometimes I walk with my sister-in-law, who is used to walking long distances and over rugged terrain. Recently we walked a local trail together. Though I hadn't distance walked in weeks, I was determined to give it my best. Unfortunately, I bought into the "no pain, no gain" myth. We walked along a dry stream bed, up steep inclines, down steep inclines, around curves, past landmarks I recognized, and then, at my request, turned around and retraced our steps. I think we walked about two miles. The next morning I could hardly move when I tried to get out of bed. All I wanted to do was groan.

What could I do? We have a charming antique tub in our bathroom. It has been resurfaced, has a hand-held shower attachment, and a book rack for lazy, soaking baths. Though I considered a warm bath, I decided against it. My legs hurt so much I didn't think I could manage to get in the tub and out again. Yikes, I could become a medical alert commercial!

The plot emerged in my mind. I pictured my husband walking in the back door and calling, "Honey, I'm home."

I could almost hear my reply. "Help, I can't get out! I'm stuck in the bathtub, the hot water is gone, I'm freezing, and wrinkled as a prune." Getting stuck in the tub because of my foolishness would be so embarrassing. The moral of this fictional scene is to return to your walking program gradually, and increase your distance each day. So please use the following pages.

Walking Log Form

Date   Weather   #Steps   Observations

_____

_____

_____

_____

_____

_____

_____

_____

_____

_____

_____

_____

_____

_____

_____

_____

_____

_____

_____

_____

_____

_____

_____

Walking Log, continued

Quotes

Searching for these quotes was fun. Some will make you smile, some will make you think, and some will make you more aware of the benefits of regular physical activity. Hopefully, others will make you laugh out loud. You may even belly laugh. I know I did when I found some of the quotes and laugh every time I read them. But many quotes are inspiring and one of my favorites is by an unknown author:

Many people will walk in and out of your life, but only true friends will leave footprints in your heart.

Friends may have left footprints in your heart at one time or another. Similarly, you may have left footprints in their hearts. Which friends have helped you most? I wouldn't be as happy as I am today were it not for a circle of friends that rallied to help me. Though I haven't seen them very much in the last year, I know these friends are still supportive.

Think about yourself and your friends while you are reading these quotes. You may want to put checkmarks by your favorite ones. Why do you like them? What makes them meaningful? Can you apply these quotes to life? Like a musical refrain, words can stick in our minds for hours and days. These words from famous and unknown people are intended to keep you moving. Walking will help your outlook and your heart.

Quotes

If I have to, I can do anything. I am strong, I am invincible, I am Woman.

Helen Reddy

I define comfort as self-acceptance when we finally learn that self-care begins and ends with ourselves.

Jennifer Louden

No trumpets sound when the important decisions of our life are made. Destiny is made known silently.

Agnes De Mille

If you exercise on a regular basis, you will have more energy.

Robert Veninga, MD

It is very important to have the right clothing to exercise in. If you throw on an old t-shirt or sweats, it's not inspiring for your workout.

Cheryl Tiegs

Between saying and doing many a pair of shoes is worn out.

Italian Proverb

Walking Woman

The human body was designed to walk, run or stop; it wasn't built for coasting.

Cullen Hightower

We can do anything we want as long as we stick to it long enough.

Helen Keller

Action is eloquence.

William Shakespeare

The distance is nothing; it's only the first step that is difficult.

Marquise du Deffand

I travel not to go anywhere, but to go.

Robert Louis Stevenson

There are only two options regarding commitment. You're either IN or you're OUT. There's no such thing as a life in-between.

Pat Riley

Quotes

For there is no friend like a sister in calm or stormy weather; To cheer one on the tedious way, to fetch if one goes astray, to lift if one totters down, to strengthen whilst one stands.

Christina Rossetti

It's important to remember that feminism is no longer a group of organizations or leaders. It's the expectations that parents have for their daughters, and their sons, too. It's the way we talk about and treat one another. It's who made the money and who makes the compromises and who makes the dinner. It's a state of mind. It's the way we live now.

Anna Quindlen

The contented person enjoys the scenery of a detour.

Author Unknown.

She who travels grubbiest travels light.

Erma Bombeck

Never journey without something to eat in your pocket. If only to throw to dogs when attacked by them.

E.S. Bates

Lack of exercise destroys the good condition of every human being, while movement and methodical physical exercise save it and preserve it.

Plato

Walking Woman

The major barriers people face when trying to increase physical activity are time, access to convenient facilities, and safe environment in which to be active.

President's Council on Physical Fitness and Sports

I will walk regularly for my soul and my body tags along.

Sarah Breathnach

Walking has been one of the constellations in the starry sky of human culture, a constellation whose three stars are the body, the imagination, and the wide-open world.

Rebecca Solnit

I'm in shape. Round is a shape . . . isn't it?

Author Unknown

A pinch of probability is worth a pound of perhaps.

James Thurber

To eat is a necessity, but to eat intelligently is an art.

La Rochefoucauld

Quotes

I love milk so much. I make a point of drinking a glass of milk every day.

Natalie Portman

Golf is a good walk spoiled.

Mark Twain

I wanted to be the first woman to burn her bra, but it would have taken the fire department four days to put it out.

Dolly Parton

Sisterhood is powerful.

Robin Morgan

The dreamer and the dream are the same . . . the powers personified in a dream are those that move the world.

Joseph Campbell

If you tell enough people what you're doing, you'll find someone who will want to help.

Michelle Sturm

Walking Woman

Never eat more than you can lift.

Miss Piggy

*A man's [or woman's] health can be judged by which he takes two at a time –
pills or stairs.*

Joan Welsh

*People say that losing weight is no walk in the park. When I hear that I think,
yeah, that's the problem.*

Chris Adams

Fitness – If it came in a bottle, everybody would have a great body.

Cher

*You start out happy that you have no hips or boobs. All of a sudden you get them,
and it feels sloppy. Then just when you start liking them, they start drooping.*

Cindy Crawford

*Volumes are now being written and spoken about the effect of the mind on the
body – I wish more was thought of the effect of the body on the mind.*

Florence Nightengale

Quotes

A vigorous five-mile walk will do more good for an unhappy but otherwise healthy adult than all the medicine and psychology in the world.

Paul Dudley White

Little by little one walks far.

Peruvian Proverb

You have to keep moving. My grandmother started walking five miles a day when she was sixty. She's ninety-three today and we don't know where the hell she is.

Ellen de Generes

Many people believe that dealing with overweight and obesity is a personal responsibility. To some degree they are right, but it is also a community responsibility. Where there are no safe, accessible places for children to play or adults to walk, job, or ride a bike, that is a community responsibility.

David Satcher, MD

To know the road ahead, ask those coming back.

Proverb

You have to be careful if you don't know where you are going, because you might not get there.

Yogi Berra

Walking Woman

Exercise and application produce order in our affairs, health of body, cheerfulness of mind, and these make us precious to our friends.

Thomas Jefferson

The body of a man [or woman] is a machine which winds its own springs.

J.O. de La Mettrie

The only way I'd worry about the weather is if it snows on our side of the field and not on theirs.

Tommy Lasorda

I figure practice puts brains in your muscles.

Sam Snead

Two roads diverged in a yellow wood, And sorry I could not travel both.

Robert Frost

It is a great art to saunter.

Henry David Thoroeau

Quotes

There is a lot more juice in grapefruit than meets the eye.

Author Unknown

I've been noticing gravity since I was young.

Cameron Diaz

If I knew I was going to live this long, I'd have taken better care of myself.

Mickey Mantle

Challenges make you discover things about yourself that you never really knew.

Cecily Tyson

Sport is a preserver of health.

Hippocrates

Everyone has limits on the time they can devote to exercise, and cross training simply gives you the best return on your investment.

Paula Newby-Fraser

Walking Woman

At a certain level, success is determined by mental factors, by dedication and motivation, and these things can't be faked. You either really care or you don't.

Arnold Schwarzenegger

The longest journey begins with a single step.

Lau Tsu

Today I have grown taller from walking with the trees.

Karle Wilson Baker

There is nothing like walking to get the feel of a country. A fine landscape is like a piece of music; it must be taken at the right tempo.

Paul Scott Mower

All happiness depends on a leisurely breakfast.

John Gunther

To drink is human, to drink coffee is divine.

Author Unknown

Quotes

Everywhere is within walking distance if you have the time.

Steven Wright

If you want to know if your brain is flabby, feel your legs.

Bruce Barton

All truly great thoughts are conceived by walking.

Frederick Nietzsche

To feel fit as a fiddle you must tone down your middle.

Author Unknown

You have to expect things of yourself before you can do them.

Michael Jordan

The place where you lose the trail is not necessarily the place where it ends.

Tom Brown, Jr.

Walking Woman

Many people will walk in and out of your life, but only true friends will leave footprints in your heart.

Author Unknown

Never have a path for walking less than three feet wide.

Martin Hoyles

Our way is not soft grass, it's a mountain path with lots of rocks. But it goes upward, forward, toward the sun.

Ruth Westheimer

When one has tasted watermelon he [or she] knows what angels eat.

Mark Twain

If you wait, all that happens is that you get older.

Larry McMurty

The longer I work in nutrition, the more convinced I become that for the healthy person all foods should be delicious.

Adele Davis

Quotes

There's something wrong with a society that drives a car to work out in a gym.

Bill Nye

Take nothing for granted. Not one blessed, cool mountain day or one hellish, desert day or one sweaty, stinky, hiking companion. It is all a gift.

Cindy Ross

Dear Lord, if you pick 'em up, I'll put 'em down.

Hiker's Prayer

Nature and I are two.

Woody Allen

Do not tread, mosey, hop, trample, step, plod, tip-toe, trot, traipse, meander, creep, prance, amble, jog, trudge, march, stomp, toddle, jump, stumble, trod, sprint, or walk on the plants.

Sign at Mount Ranier National Park

My father considered a walk among the mountains as the equivalent of church-going.

Aldos Huxley

Walking Woman

In every walk with nature one receives far more than he seeks.

John Muir

Walking with a friend in the dark is better than walking alone at night.

Helen Keller

Don't compromise yourself. You are all you've got.

Janis Joplin

Don't knock the weather: nine tenths of the people couldn't start a conversation if it didn't change once in a while.

Kim Hubbard

We sit at breakfast, we sit on the train on the way to work, we sit at work, we sit at lunch, we sit all afternoon, a hodgepodge of sagging livers, sinking gall bladders, drooping stomachs, compressed intestines, and squashed pelvic organs.

John Button, Jr.

Walking is the best possible exercise.

Thomas Jefferson

Quotes

If it weren't for the fact that the TV set and the refrigerator are so far apart, some of us wouldn't get any exercise at all.

Joey Adams

Those who think they have not time for bodily exercise will sooner or later have to find time for illness.

Edward Stanley

Scatter poems on the floor; Turn the poet out of door.

Robert Frost

There is no easy way out [of exercise]. If there were, I would have bought it. And believe me, it would be one of my favorite things!

Oprah Winfrey

There is delight, too, in the physical fitness that comes only after weeks and weeks of walking. The body works at its best when used every day, and the feeling this gives is tremendous.

Chris Townsend

A birthday is just the first day of another 365-day journey around the sun. Enjoy the trip.

Author Unknown

Walking Woman

I dream of hiking into my old age. I want to be able even then to pack my load and take off slowly but steadily along the trail.

Marlyn Doan

Even the woodpecker owes his success to the fact that he uses his head and keeps pecking away until he finishes the job he starts.

Coleman Cox

The Centers for Disease Control and Prevention [CDC] estimates that a difference of 100 calories of exercise per person per day, the equivalent of 20 minutes of walking, could eliminate the obesity epidemic we are now experiencing.

Michael P. O'Donnell

If you can't be a good example, then you'll just have to be a horrible warning.

Catherine Aird

You must think of yourself as becoming the person you want to be.

David Viscott

I can remember walking as a child. It was not customary to say you were fatigued. It was customary to complete the goal of the expedition.

Katharine Hepburn

Quotes

Don't walk in front of me, I may not follow. Don't walk behind me, I may not lead. Walk beside me and be my friend.

Albert Camus

One step at a time is good walking.

Chinese Proverb

Rich, fatty foods are like destiny; they too, shape our ends.

Author Unknown

Life itself is the proper binge.

Julia Child

Every day you make progress. Every step may be fruitful. Yet there will stretch out before you an ever-lengthening, ever-ascending, ever-improving path. You know you will never get to the end of the journey. But this, so far from discouraging, only adds to the joy and glory of the climb.

Sir Winston Churchill

Climb the mountains and get their good tidings. Nature's peace will flow into you as sunshine flows into trees. The winds will blow their freshness into you, and the storms their energy, while cares will drop like falling leaves.

John Muir

Walking Woman

To love oneself is the beginning of a lifelong romance.

Oscar Wilde

The greatest discovery of my generation is that human beings can alter their lives by altering their attitude of mind.

William James

Enthusiasm is contagious. Start an epidemic.

Don Ward

Birthdays are good for you. Statistics show that the people who have the most live the longest.

Larry Lorenzoni

If we did all the things we were capable of doing, we would literally astound ourselves.

Thomas Edison

My passport photo is one of the most remarkable photographs I have ever seen – no retouching, no shadows, no flattery – just stark me

Anne Morrow Lindbergh

Quotes

Aerodynamically, the bumblebee shouldn't be able to fly, but the bumblebee doesn't know it so it goes on flying anyway.

Mary Kay Ash

Thirty to sixty minutes of activity broken into smaller segments of 15 minutes throughout the day has significant health benefits.

President's Council on Physical Fitness and Sports

It's always too soon to quit!

Norman Vincent Peale

Some people like to make a little garden out of life and walk down a path.

Jan Anouilh

Tell me what you eat and I will tell you what you are.

Anita Brookner

Want to learn to eat a lot? Here it is: Eat a little. That way, you'll be around long enough to eat a lot.

Anthony Robbins

Walking Woman

Self delusion is pulling in your stomach when you step on the scale.

Paul Sweeny

Chairlifts are needed so we can get to the wonderful views without having to hike them.

Comment received by the U.S. Forest Service

Hiking a ridge, a meadow, a river bottom, is as healthy a form of exercise as one can get.

William O. Douglas

It's hard to beat a person who never gives up.

Babe Ruth

Before supper take a little walk, after supper do the same.

Erasmus

You've heard this before, my friend, but I have to say it again because this is my last chance to say it. You're not going out there to prove anything. You're not going out there to rough it. You're going out there to smooth it. You get it rough enough every day!

Harry Roberts

Quotes

We are under-exercised as a nation. We look instead of play. We ride instead of walk. Our existence deprives us of the minimum of physical activity essential to healthy living.

John F. Kennedy

If you aren't going all the way, why go at all?

Joe Namath

Most people are pantywaists. Exercise is good for you.

Emma Gatewood

I'm a slow walker, but I never walk backwards.

Abraham Lincoln

If we're not willing to settle for junk living, we certainly shouldn't settle for junk food.

Sally Edwards

Your stomach shouldn't be a waste basket.

Author Unknown

Walking Woman

*Get action. Seize the moment. Man [or woman] was never intended to become
an oyster.*

Theodore Roosevelt

Even if you are on the right track, you'll get run over if you just sit there.

Will Rogers

My body is a sacred garment.

Martha Graham

Happiness consists in activity. It is a running stream not a stagnant pool.

John Mason Good

Water is the only drink for a wise man [or woman].

Henry David Thoreau

There are no short cuts to any place worth going.

Beverly Sills

Quotes

A man [or woman] too busy to take care of his health is like a mechanic too busy to take care of his tools.

Spanish Proverb

The sole criteria is to walk with the senses, with hands that feel, ears that hear, and eyes that see.

Robert Browne

Too great talkers will not travel far together.

George Borrow

Exercise should be fun, otherwise, you won't be consistent.

Laura Ramirez

Slow down and enjoy life. It's not only the scenery you miss by going fast – you also miss the sense of where you are going and why.

Eddie Cantor

I come from a family where gravy is considered a beverage.

Erma Bombeck

Walking Woman

Young at heart. Slightly older in other places.

Author Unknown

Life is very interesting . . . in the end, some of your greatest pains become your greatest strengths.

Drew Barrymore

People usually consider walking on water or in thin air as a miracle. But I think the real miracle is not to walk either on water or in the air, but to walk on earth.

Thich Nhat Hanh

All walking is discovery. On foot we take the time to see things whole.

Hal Borland

A McDonald's would be nice at trailhead.

Comment received by the US Forest Service

As the life of the horse is in his legs, so the life of the traveler is in his [or her] feet, and good care should be taken of them.

Juliette de Bairacli Levy

Quotes

You're not obligated to win. You're obligated to keep trying and to do the best you can every day.

Marian Wright Edelman

Physical activity is an excellent stress-buster and provides other health benefits as well. It can also improve your mood and image.

Jon Wickham

The value of a principle is the number of things it will explain.

Ralph Waldo Emerson

Gardening is a great way to not only connect with nature, but to take advantage of the health benefits you can rake in as well.

Kelly Haugen

If you want a place in the sun you've got to put up with a few blisters.

Abigail Van Buren

Take a two-mile walk before breakfast.

Harry Truman

Walking Woman

Sunshine is delicious, rain is refreshing, wind braces up, snow is exhilarating; there is no such thing as bad weather just different kinds of good weather.

John Ruskin

There is no challenge more challenging than the challenge to improve yourself.

Michael F. Staley

A willing heart adds feather to the heel.

Joanna Baillie

It's a very slow process – two steps forward, one step back – but I'm inching in the right direction.

Rob Reiner

Good walking leaves no track behind it.

Lau Tsu

It may be possible to incorporate laughter into daily activities, just as is done with other heart-healthy activities, such as taking the stairs instead of the elevator. The recommendation for a healthy heart may one day be exercise, eat right and laugh a few times a day.

Michael Miller, MD

Quotes

You don't take a photograph, you make it.

Ansel Adams

Whoever thought up the word "Mammogram?" Every time I hear it I think I'm supposed to put my breast in an envelope and send it to someone.

Jan King

The greatest thing in the world is not so much where we are, but in which direction we are moving.

Oliver Wendell Holmes

Life is a series of steps. Things are done gradually. Once in a while there is a giant step, but most of the time we are taking small, seemingly insignificant steps on the stairway of life.

Ralph Ransom

One should eat to live, not live to eat.

Benjamin Franklin

My grandmother is over eighty and still doesn't need glasses. Drinks right out of the bottle.

Henny Youngman

Walking Woman

In order to change we must be sick and tired of being sick and tired.

Author Unknown

How glorious a greeting the sun gives the mountains.

John Muir

We all get heavier as we get older because there's lots more information in our heads.

Valde Divac

We must walk before we run.

George Barrow

There is this to be said for walking: It's the one mode of human locomotion by which a man [or woman] proceeds on his [or her] own two feet, upright, erect, as a man [or woman] should be, not squatting on his rear haunches like a frog.

Edward Abbey

Another belief of mine: that everyone else my age is an adult, whereas I am merely in disguise.

Margaret Atwood

Quotes

When you have worn out your shoes, the strength of the shoe leather has passed into the fiber of your body. I measure your health by the number of shoes and hats and clothes you have worn out.

Ralph Waldo Emerson

He who does not mind his belly will hardly mind anything else.

Samuel Johnson

Big doesn't necessarily mean better. Sunflowers aren't better than violets.

Edna Ferber

Never lend your car to anyone to whom you have given birth.

Erma Bombeck

Take care of your body with steadfast fidelity. The soul must see through these eyes alone, and if they are dim, the whole world is clouded.

Johann Wolfgang Von Goethe

I made my way downstairs. The stairs lead the way down onto the . . . street. They lead all the way up too, of course . . . saves me having two stairways.

Chic Murray

Walking Woman

We keep moving forward, opening new doors, and doing new things because we're curious and curiosity keeps leading us down new paths.

Walt Disney

Beauty is in the eye of the beholder and it may be necessary from time to time to give a stupid or misinformed beholder a black eye.

Miss Piggy

To lengthen your life shorten your meals.

Proverb

Get on your horse, mule, bicycle or feet, and come on in. Enjoy yourselves. This here park is for people.

Edward Abbey

Physical fitness is vital for the optimal function of the brain, for retardation of the onset of serious arteriosclerosis which is beginning to appear in early adult life, and for longevity, and a useful and healthy life for older citizens.

Paul Dudley White

Sex is good, but not as good as fresh sweet corn

Garrison Keillor

Quotes

You must take action now that will move you towards your goals. Develop a sense of urgency in your life.

Les Brown

I'm not afraid of storms, for I'm learning to sail my ship.

Louisa May Alcott

Trust only movement. Life happens at the level of events, not of words. Trust movement.

Alfred Adler

The vision must be followed by the venture. It is not enough to start up the steps – we must step up the stairs.

Vance Havner

Television has changed a child from an irresistible force to an immovable object.

Author Unknown

Food is an important part of a balanced diet.

Fran Lebowitz

Walking Woman

Well begun is half done.

Aristotle

Keep on going, and the chances are that you will stumble on something, perhaps when you are least expecting it. I never heard of anyone stumbling on something sitting down.

Charles F. Kettering

All God's children need traveling shoes.

Maya Angelou

Don't be discouraged. It's often the last key in the bunch that opens the lock.

Author Unknown

A handful of pine-seed will cover mountains with the green majesty of forest. I will set my face to the wind and throw my handful of seed on high.

Fiona Macleod

Sons branch out, but one woman leads to another.

Margaret Atwood

Quotes

There is no more creative force in the world than the menopausal woman with zest.

Margaret Mead

A rainy day is the perfect time for a walk in the woods.

Rachael Carson

Smokers who blow smoke in my face will learn firsthand (within minutes actually) how injurious smoking can be to their health.

Erma Bombeck

I frequently tramped eight or ten miles through the deepest snow to keep an appointment with a birch-tree, or yellow birch, or an old acquaintance among the pines.

Henry David Thoreau

All people are made alike – of bones and flesh and dinner. Only the dinners are different.

Gertrude Louise Cheney

Perseverance is the hard work you do after you get tired of doing the hard work you already did.

Newt Gingrich

Walking Woman

There is an expression – walking with beauty. And I believe that this endless search for beauty in surroundings, in people and one's personal life, is the headstone of travel.

Juliette De Bairacli Levy

I've been chasing rainbows since I was a kid, Seekin' out the paths where no others did.

Walkin' Jim Stolz

I have gained and lost the same ten pounds so many times over and over again my cellulite must have déjà vu.

Jane Wagner

I love the challenge.

Nancy Lopez

Keep your face to the sunshine and you cannot see a shadow.

Helen Keller

It takes a very long time to become young.

Pablo Picasso

Quotes

Simplifying your life gives you more time for what you really do want time and energy for (like exercising, or reading, or taking a class).

Kathy Gates

If we are facing in the right direction, all we have to do is keep on walking.

Buddhist Saying

Walking would teach people the quality that youngsters find so hard to learn – patience.

Edward P. Weston

Health is a state of complete physical, mental and social well-being, and not merely the absence of disease or infirmity.

World Health Organization

And what exactly is nature walking? It's any and every kind of walking you can do in the natural world. The activity encompasses strolling, striding, sauntering, stepping, treading, tramping, traipsing, traversing, rambling, roving, roaming, racewalking, hiking, meandering, wandering, wending, pacing, peregrinating, perambulating.

Charles Cook

Running [or walking] is the greatest metaphor for life, because you get out of it what you put into it.

Oprah Winfrey

Walking Woman

Life is uncertain. Eat dessert first.

Ernestine Ulmer

The first step towards getting somewhere is to decide that you are not going to stay where you are.

John Pierpont Morgan

I have often started off on a walk in the state called mad – mad in the sense of sore-headed, or mad with tedium or confusion; I have set forth dull, null and even thoroughly discouraged. But I never came back in such a frame of mind, and I never met a human being whose humor was not the better for a walk.

Donald Culcross Peattie

Help one another is part of the religion of sisterhood.

Louisa May Alcott

I have to exercise in the morning before my brain figures out what I'm doing.

Marsha Doble

I represent what is left of a vanishing race, and that is the pedestrian . . . That I am still able to be here, I owe to a keen eye and a nimble pair of legs. But I know they'll get me someday.

Will Rogers

Quotes

Leave the beaten track occasionally and dive into the woods. Every time you do so you will be certain to find something that you have never seen before.
Alexander Graham Bell

Trails need to be reconstructed. Please avoid building trails that go uphill.
Comment received by the US Forest Service

We load up on oat bran in the morning. Then we spend the rest of the day living like there's no tomorrow.
Lee Iacocca

An idea not coupled with action will never get any bigger than the brain cell it occupied.
Arnold Glasgow

If you are seeking creative ideas, go out walking. Angels whisper to a man [or woman] when he [she] goes for a walk.
Raymond Inmon

If high heels were so wonderful, men would still be wearing them.
Sue Grafton

Walking Woman

Our bodies are molded in rivers.

Norvalis

I really don't think I need buns of steel. I'd be happy with buns of cinnamon.
Ellen DeGeneres

To enjoy city walking to the utmost you have to throw yourself into a mood of loving humanity.

Donald Culross Peattie

When you come to a fork in the road take it.

Yogi Berra

Few actions can do more to make urban areas safer, healthier, prettier, and more environmentally balanced than setting aside corridors or trails for walking, biking, wildlife watching, and just plain breaking up the monotony of cars and concrete.

James Snyder

Sleep is the golden chain that ties health and our bodies together.
Thomas Dekker

Quotes

In general my children refuse to eat anything that hasn't danced on television.
Erma Bombeck

The secret of staying young is to live honestly, eat slowly, and lie about your age.
Lucille Ball

I only went for a walk, and finally concluded to stay out till sundown, for going out, I found, was really going in.
John Muir

I am a verb.
Ulysses S. Grant

Many a false step is made standing still.
Pattie Labelle

It's like the code of living by yourself. People who are single know what I'm talking about. You eat standing up, reading the paper.
Mary C. Carpenter

Walking Woman

Learn the art of patience. Apply discipline to your thoughts when they become anxious over the outcome of a goal. Impatience breeds anxiety, fear, discouragement and failure. Patience creates confidence, decisiveness, and a rational outlook, which eventually leads to success.

Brian Adams

Far away there in the sunshine are my highest aspirations. I may not reach them, but I can look up and see their beauty, believe in them, and try to follow where they lead.

Louisa May Alcott

We are what we repeatedly do.

Aristotle

Right here and now, moving through space on my own two strong legs, I am meditating. Each breath I breathe is in tune with the morning.

Bettyclare Moffatt

As long as I can walk and talk I'll try almost anything. I say "almost" because the high wire is definitely out.

Lauren Bacall

The Outdoor Recreation Resources Commission marked a notable point . . . The simple, close-to-home activities, it discovered, are by and far away the most important to Americans. . . The structure of our metropolitan areas has long since been set by nature and man, by the rivers and hills, and the railroads and highways. Many options remain, and the great task of planning is not to come up with another structure but to work within the strengths we have.

William Whyte

Quotes

Every path has its puddle.

English Proverb

The path to our destination is not always a straight one. We go down the wrong road, we get lost, we turn back. Maybe it doesn't matter which road we embark on. Maybe what matters is that we embark.

Barbara Hall

Everything we do seeds the future. No action is an empty one.

Joan Chittister

Here's the typical evolution I see in so many people when they first begin a regular aerobic program. Initially, they are happily surprised to see inches leave their body. Next, they're excited about new-found energy reserves. And then they're inspired to add a third and fourth day of aerobic activity, even something as simple as walking.

Jacki Sorensen

I'm not going to vacuum til Sears makes one you can ride on.

Roseanne Barr

Success is not a destination that you ever reach. Success is the quality of your journey.

Jennifer James

Walking Woman

Keep your eye fixed on the path to the top, but don't forget to look right in front of you. The last step depends on the first.

Rene Daumal

Great walking cities are those with destinations within a 15-to-20 minute walk of each other . . . varied architecture. Diverse neighborhoods with a lively street life energized by sidewalk vendors, entertainers, and window-shoppers . . . filled with open spaces and parks . . . widened with sidewalks, auto-restricted zones, and ameneties such as benches, signs and fountains.

Walking Magazine

Never accept a drink from a Urologist.

Erma Bombeck

The mosquito is the state bird of New Jersey.

Andy Warhol

[Walking's] overwhelming advantage is that it can be done by anyone, anytime, anywhere – and it doesn't even look like exercise.

Kenneth H. Cooper, MD

Sometime in your life you will go on a journey. It will be the longest journey you have ever taken. It is the journey to find yourself.

Katherine Sharp

Quotes

The minute you settle for less than you deserve, you get even less than you settled for.

Maureen Dowd

Movement is in your nature – put it in your routine.

Mark Fenton

The body says what words cannot.

Martha Graham

Grab your coat, and get your hat, Leave your worry at the doorstep.

Dorothy Fields

Begin doing what you want to do now. We are not living in eternity. We only have this moment, sparkling like a star in our hand.

Marie Beyon

Time is a dressmaker specializing in alterations.

Faith Baldwin

Walking Woman

We don't know who we are until we see what we can do.

Martha Grimes

Our deeds determine us, as much as we determine our deeds.

George Eliot

Leave the table while you still feel you could eat a little more.

Helena Rubenstein

Television is an instrument which can paralyze this country.

General William C. Westmoreland

The Moon Pie is a bedrock of the country store and rural tradition. It is more than a snack. It is a cultural artifact.

William Ferris

I wake up in the morning, I do a little stretching exercises, pick up the horn and play.

Herb Alpert

Quotes

Keep busy while you are waiting for something to happen.

Robert Genn

I don't diet. I just don't eat as much as I'd like to.

Linda Evangelista

I wave my hat to all I see, and they wave back to me.

Jim Stolz

The soles on my shoes were so thin I could step on a coin and tell if it was heads or tails.

Tommy Lasorda

Take care of your body. It's the only place you have to live.

Jim Rohn

What I must do is all that concerns me, not what the people think.

Ralph Waldo Emerson

Walking Woman

Put a grain of boldness in everything you do.

Baltasar Gracian

I think stretching before training and the match has helped me, as well as being sensible with my eating and drinking.

Richard Gough

Good friends are good for your health.

Irwin Sarason

The future belongs to those who believe in the beauty of their dreams.

Eleanor Roosevelt

The preservation of health is a duty. Few seem conscious that there is such a thing as physical morality.

Herbert Spencer

A balanced diet is a cookie in each hand.

Author Unknown

Quotes

More die in the United States of too much food than too little.

John Kenneth Galbraith

Take it with a grin of salt.

Yogi Berra

And in the end, it's not the years in your life that count. It's the life in your years.

Abraham Lincoln

We can't all be great explorers, like Perry and Powell, nor great naturalists, like Thoreau and Humboldt. But anyone who prizes the sights and sounds of nature in action, whether robins at the window or muskrat in the stream, or a bog born of ages, such a one is, within his [or her] measure, an explorer and naturalist.

Benton MacKaye

So much has been said and sung of beautiful young girls, why don't somebody wake up to the beauty of old women.

Harriet Beecher Stowe

It is difficult to stop [painting] in time because one gets carried away. But I have that strength, it is the only one I have.

Claude Monet

Walking Woman

Teamwork: Simply stated, it is less me and more we.

Author Unknown

You can only hold in your stomach for so many years.

Burt Reynolds

Oh, my dear, it's a buffet. I have chicken a la king. I have cold turkey. I have hot rolls. I have cold ham. I have a big watermelon, all filled with fresh fruits.

Perle Mesta

The trouble is that humans do have a knack for choosing precisely those things that are worst for them.

J.K. Rowling

Why walk? Because it makes you feel good and makes you look good.

John Man

Change, like sunshine, can be a friend or a foe, a blessing or a curse, a dawn or a dusk.

William A. Ward

Quotes

It is easy to live for others; everybody does. I call on you to live for yourselves.

Ralph Waldo Emerson

One is not born a woman, one becomes one.

Simone de Beauvoir

The inescapable duty to observe oneself; if someone else is observing me, naturally I have to observe myself too; if none observe me, I have to observe myself all the closer.

Franz Kafka

I don't wait for moods. You accomplish nothing if you do that. Your mind must know it has to get down to work.

Pearl Buck

I am a woman above everything else.

Jacqueline Kennedy

Teamwork doesn't tolerate the inconvenience of distance.

Author Unknown.

Walking Woman

I like vending machines because snacks are better when they fall. If I buy a candy bar at the store oftentimes I will drop it, so that it achieves its maximum flavor potential.

Mitch Hedberg

Patience serves as protection against wrongs as clothes do against cold. For if you put on more clothes as the cold increases, it will have no power to hurt you. So in like manner you must grow in patience when you meet with great wrongs, and they will then be powerless to vex your mind.

Leonardo da Vinci

Too many bugs and leeches and spiders and spider webs. Please spray the wilderness to rid area of these pests.

Comment received by the U.S. Forest Service

Motivation is what gets you started. Habit is what keeps you going.

Jim Rohn

You have a choice. It may not be a choice you like, but it's still a choice.

Michelle Pfeiffer

I like to walk amidst the beautiful things that adorn the world.

George Santayana

Quotes

It is remarkable how one's wits are sharpened by physical exercise.

Pliny the Younger

We live in a fast-paced society. Walking slows us down.

Robert Sweetgall

You're not 40, you're 18 with 22 years of experience.

Author Unknown

Opportunities are often things you haven't noticed the first time around.

Catherine Deneuve

Muscles come and go; flab lasts.

Bill Vaughan

The word aerobic comes from two Greek words: aero, meaning "ability to," and bics, meaning "withstand tremendous boredom."

Dave Berry

Walking Woman

Walking your talk is a great way to motivate yourself. No one likes to live a lie. Be honest with yourself and you will find the motivation to do what you advise others to do.

Vince Posconte

I can't be funny if my feet don't feel right.

Billy Crystal

You don't need a fancy-schmancy treadmill.

James Levine, MD

Exercise while watching your favorite TV show.

Michael Lee

I always recommend a sensible diet, including lots of carbohydrates and avoiding too much fat. Dancers don't need different fuel from other people – they just need more of it because they use more energy.

Deborah Bull

I believe a leaf of grass is no less than the journey-work of the stars.

Walt Whitman

Quotes

The American people never carry an umbrella. They are prepared to walk in eternal sunshine.

Alfred E. Smith

Nature abhors a vacuum, and if I can only walk with sufficient carelessness I am sure to be filled.

Henry David Thoreau

Exercise should be regarded as tribute to the heart.

Gene Tunney

For you, as well as I, can open fence doors and walk across America in your own special way. Then we can all discover who our neighbors are.

Rob Sweetgall

I'm not overweight. I'm just nine inches too short.

Shelly Winters

To me a lush carpet of pine needles or spongy grass is more welcome than the most luxurious Persian rug.

Helen Keller

Walking Woman

Parents can only give good advice or put them [children] on the right paths, but the final forming of a person's character lies in their own hands.

Anne Frank

Ambition is a dream with a V-8 engine.

Elvis Presley

Remember, Ginger Rogers did everything Fred Astaire did, but she did it backwards and in high heels.

Faith Whittlesey

When I find myself fading, I close my eyes and realize my friends are my energy.

Author Unknown

None of us is as smart as all of us.

Ken Blanchard

Use it or lose it.

Jimmy Connors

Quotes

October is a symphony of permanence and change.

Author Unknown

Success in walking is not to let your right foot know what your left foot doeth. Your heart must furnish such music that in keeping time to it your feet will carry you around the globe without knowing it.

John Burroughs

An early morning walk is a blessing for the whole day.

Henry David Thoreau

A diet is when you watch what you eat and wish you could eat what you watch.

Hermione Gingold

My wife and I eat out practically every night, and I've got every restaurant trained. The Chinese restaurants we go to have brown rice, and other restaurants make sure they have the right soups for us, with no butter or cream.

Jack LaLanne

I take vitamins daily, but just the bare essentials, not what you'd call supplements.

Clint Eastwood

Walking Woman

You are never given a wish without also being given the power to make it come true. You may have to work for it, however.

Richard Bach

Self-knowledge is the beginning of self-improvement.

Spanish Proverb

May your stuffing be tasty
May your turkey be plump.
May your potatoes and gravy
Have nary a lump.
May your yams be delicious
And your pies take the prize.
And may your Thanksgiving dinner
Stay off your thighs!

Author Unknown

Seize the moment. Remember all those women on the Titanic who waived off the dessert cart.

Erma Bombeck

Obstacles are those frightening things that become visible when we take our eyes off our goals.

Henry Ford

If you train hard, you'll not only be hard, you'll be hard to beat.

Herschel Walker

Quotes

Train, don't strain.

Arthur Lydiard

Saying no can be the ultimate self care.

Claudia Black

Make your feet your friend.

J.M. Barrie

Technique isn't enough on its own – emotion has to come through – but when you've got technique sewn up, that's one thing you don't have to worry about.

Zoe Benbow

Over the years our bodies become walking autobiographies, telling friends and strangers alike of the minor and major stresses of our lives.

Marilyn Ferguson

Ninety percent of the game is half mental.

Yogi Berra

Walking Woman

Your success as a family, our success as a society, depends not on what happens in the White House, but what happens inside your house.

Barbara Bush

I still need more healthy rest in order to work at my best. My health is the main capital and I want to administer it intelligently.

Ernest Hemingway

I have outwalked the furthest city light.

Robert Frost

A committee of one gets things done.

Joe Ryan

Walking companions, like heroes, are difficult to pluck out of the crowd of acquaintances. Good dispositions, ready wit, friendly conversation serve well enough by the fireside but they prove insufficient in the field. For there you need transcendentalists – nothing less; you need poets, sages, humorists and natural philosophers.

Brooke Atkinson

Afoot and light-hearted, I take to the open road, Healthy, free, the world before me.

Walt Whitman

Quotes

There is no orthodoxy in walking. It is a land of many paths and no-paths.

George Maculay Trevelyn

Above all, do not lose your desire to walk. Every day I walk myself into a state of well-being and walk away from every illness. I have walked myself into my best thoughts, and I know of no thought so burdensome that one cannot walk away from it . . . if one just keeps on walking, everything will be all right.

Soren Kierkegaard

Thank you for calling the Weight Loss Hotline. If you'd like to lose half a pound right now, press one eighteen thousand times.

Author Unknown

Never ride when you can walk.

Bill Gale

Trails in the 21st century will be characterized by meaningful connections, whereby all Americans will have access to parks, places of employment, and neighboring communities.

12th National Trails Symposium

Walk and be happy, walk and be healthy. The best way to lengthen out our days is to walk steadily and with a purpose.

Charles Dickens

Walking Woman

Kissing don't last; cookery do!

George Meredith

I've really never accepted the idea that a woman can't do whatever the hell it is she wants.

Sylvia Chase

You can set yourself out to be sick, or you can choose to stay well.

Wayne Dyer

Trails need to be wider so people can walk holding hands.

Comment received by the U.S. Forest Service

A sister is a gift to the heart, a friend to the spirit, a golden thread to the meaning of life.

Isadora James

To exist is to change, to change is to mature, to mature is to go on creating oneself endlessly.

Henri Bergson

Quotes

Coming together, sharing together, working together, succeeding together.

Author Unknown

If you look deeply into the palm of your hand, you will see your parents and all generations of your ancestors.

Thich Nhat Hanh

There is no telling how many miles you have to run [or walk] while chasing a dream.

Author Unknown

May you always walk with sunshine. May you never want for more. May Irish angels rest their wings right beside your door.

Irish Blessing

Some Final Thoughts

You may be wondering if there is an ending to my health story. Well, there is an ending of sorts. My primary care physician ordered tests for me, an echocardiogram, electrocardiogram, and special blood tests. She also referred me to a cardiologist. During the echocardiogram I admit to having worrisome thoughts as I listened to the "woosha, woosha, woosha" of my leaking valve. My worry increased when the technician left to get a cardiologist and told me not to worry.

How could I not worry? A few days earlier my husband commented, "I think hearing my heart beats is reassuring. Do you?"

"No," I answered. "I'm afraid the woosha sound will become clanka-clanka."

As I have aged my defective heart valve has become stiffer and this allows more blood to flow in the wrong direction. Would I need surgery? I decided to approach surgery positively if it was recommended, trust my medical team, and focus on the future. My husband had undergone invasive surgery for me and I would do the same for him, and for those who love me.

Before I entered his office the cardiologist had reviewed my tests. He brought up the results on the computer screen so I could see them. "Your valve is still leaking," he noted, "but it's something you can live with. You can go for years with this condition, and don't need surgery." I was so relieved. Yet I am concerned about my leak staying the same and not leaking more than it is already.

My blood pressure is under control, thanks to life-saving drugs. But getting my blood pressure checked makes me anxious and I calm myself with diaphragm breathing. I've also gotten better at self-care. Turning off the television news is one of the best things I do for myself. Whether I watch or not, the news will keep happening, the newsflashes will keep coming, and I don't have to see every one.

I continue to be a walking woman and do laps in discount and megastores. To ensure regular physical activity, eliminate the hassle factor, and save on gas driving to and from stores, my husband and I bought a treadmill. It takes up a minimal amount of space, has all the features we need, and folds up. The treadmill was on sale and, thanks to a special promotion, we received a $50 cash card to use in the store.

After we left checkout, we drove to the loading dock to pick up our purchase. Two burly young men lifted the box and, with loud grunts, slid it into the back of our truck. The grunts should have told us something. At home, we realized the box weighed 300 pounds or more. With careful planning and coordination, we were able to slide the box out of the truck, and push it into the garage. So far, so good, but how could we get the treadmill to the lower level?

Our painter is a former gymnastics coach and weight lifter. I've had several conversations with him about fitness walking and using a treadmill. Since he was painting window frames upstairs,

I decided to approach him. "This isn't in your job description," I began, "but could you help John get the treadmill to the lower level?" He agreed instantly. We live on a hill and, to avoid two sets of stairs, the guys decided to push the box down the hill behind our house. Things started off well and then, because of the snow and the weight of the box, the treadmill began to pick up speed. How fast could it go? Would it shoot past the house, through the side lawn, and damage the neighbor's property? I could see the newspaper headline in my mind, "Runaway Treadmill Careens into Neighbor's Deck!" We would never live it down if that happened.

But the guys regained control of the box, steered it in the right direction, and stopped it in front of the patio door. My husband is a mechanical whiz and he put the treadmill together. The first time I used it my speed was two miles an hour and I walked a half hour, for a distance of one mile, pretty good for someone who hadn't used a treadmill in a while. I quickly increased this speed to 2.5 miles per hour. In less than a week, I was walking 2.7 miles an hour. Two weeks later I was walking 2.9 miles an hour. Three weeks later I was walking three miles an hour, which may be my maximum speed.

Each day I walk a mile on the treadmill. Walking has helped me lose weight and I've been losing about three-to-four pounds a month. I have a a long way to go, but at least I'm making progress. Whenever I can, wherever I can, I share my walking story. All these years, my heart has been pumping away faithfully. Now I understand (and don't know why it's taken so long for me to get this) that I can help my heart by being physically active and maintaining a healthy weight.

Before I started this book I had not heard of WomenHeart. Now I am on the email list, aware of the organization's mission, and the thousands of women it serves. Carol Allred, the Women-Heart member who wrote the back cover review, thinks of coalition members as her "heart sisters." I think of them this way, too, especially when I'm walking. Certainly these women were in my thoughts while I was writing this guide.

While you are walking think of those who walked before you – your parents, grandparents, great grandparents, and family members back in time. Think of those who walk with you – your husband, significant other, children, and grandchildren. Finally, think of those who helped make you who you are today, the family members, work colleagues, and people you've never met.

According to Native American writer and poet Linda Hogan, MA, the Chickasaw Nation Writer-in-Residence, previous generations are still with you and part of your life. In her words:

Walking, I am listening in a deeper way. Suddenly all my ancestors are behind me. Be still, they say, watch and listen. You are the result of the love of thousands.

Why does **Walking Woman** end with these thoughts? I want you to love yourself enough to take care of yourself. Much as health professionals want to help you, when you think about it, you are the best person to take care of you, and that's what this guide is about. You need to keep walking for **you** and you don't have to do it alone.

Connect with other women who are walking for heart health. According to an old saying, there is strength in numbers, and it's true. Tap this strength. Share your story with other women who are at risk for heart disease, been diagnosed with it, have had a heart attack, or are living successfully after surgery. You may not know all their names, but these women are your heart sisters, an ongoing source of support, the ones you may turn to again and again. Better yet, they understand your story, experience, and challenges.

Even if you aren't physically connected, please stay emotionally connected with your heart sisters via national conferences, phone calls, text messaging, emails, and Skype. Do you remember the time when people sent each other handwritten and typed letters? It wasn't that long ago. Send a written letter to a heart sister or several sisters. For together, you form a network of support all across America. With thousands of sisters at your side, walk your way to the future and a healthier life.

Appendix A

Helpful Websites

Websites can help you take charge of your heart disease or at risk status. While these addresses are as current as possible, as you know, they may change. Add the addresses you access most often to your computer favorites list. You may wish to pencil in additional website addresses on this page.

Health blogs may also be a source of support. Telling your story connects you with others just like you. For example, you may share your story on the WomenHeart website. You may also volunteer to be a WomenHeart Champion and knit or crochet headscarves for women. Many websites have free information you may download. Before you download anything, check the number of pages and decide if you want to spend that much on ink.

- American Heart Association, www.startwalkingnow.org
- *Arthritis Today* magazine, www.arthritistoday.org/fitness/**walking**/index.php
- BellaOnline – The Voice of Women, www.bellaonline.com/site/walking

- *California Walk Kit,* www.**ca**activecommunities.org/resources/**walk-kit**
- Calorie Count, www.carloriecount.com
- Chi**Walking,** www.chi**walking**.com
- Daily Motivation, www.50plus-fitness-**walking**.com/daily-motivatin.html
- Food Count, www.foodcount.com
- Google map pedometer, www.pedometer.com
- Map my Walk website, www.mapmywalk.com
- Mayo Clinic, www.mayoclinic.com (use the search words walking, walking benefits, fitness, aeroabic)
- MedicineNet, www.medicinenet.com/walking/article.htm
- My Calorie Counter, www.my-calorie-counter.com
- My Food Diary, www.myfooddiary.com
- My Fitness Pal, www.myfitnesspal.com
- My Walks, www.mywalks.com
- Nordic Walking Blog, www.hordicwalkingusa.blogspot.com/.../new-exel-nordic-walking-website.html
- Nutrition Data, www.nutritiondata.com
- Partnership for a Walkable America (PWA), www.wakableamerica.org
- *Prevention* magazine, www.prevention.com/fitness/fitness-tips/walking
- TAKE THE WALK, www.takethewalk.net
- The Fitness Walking Guide, www.the-fitness-walking-guide.com
- The Walking Site, www.thewalkingsite.com
- US Government, www.nutrition.gov
- Walking Connection, www.walkingconnection.com/**walking**_technique_form.html
- Walking for Fitness, www.walkingabout.com

- Wellsphere, www.wellsphere.com/viewtips.s?communityid=35
- WomenHeart, www.womanheart.org
- Women and Weight, www.womenandweight.com/reviews/calorie-counts-and-nutrients-best-sites-online/
- US Department of Transportation, www.walkinginfo.org/

Words to Know

aerobic – physical activity that causes you to use oxygen and energy more efficiently, such as speed walking, running, and swimming

aftercare – a physician-monitored program of medication, physical activity, and therapies to foster recovery

aorta – carries blood from the left side of the heart to the rest of your body

arrhythmias – irregular heartbeats

aspirin regimen – physician-managed program of daily aspirin to reduce risks of heart attack and stroke

atria – upper chambers of the heart

BMI – stands for body mass index, a calculation that helps you see if you have a healthy or unhealthy percentage of body fat; a BMI of 25 or more increases your risk of heart disease

calorie – a unit of energy measurement; to lose a pound a week you need to eat about 500 fewer calories than your body burns

cardiologist – medical doctor who specializes in heart disease

catheter – a long, flexible tube

cool down – continuing to walk slowly at the end of our walk

cholesterol – waxy substance (fats) in the blood; HDL is the "good" cholesterol, LDL is the "bad" and clogs arteries

cross-training – using different types of physical activities to become fit

daily calorie burn – number of calories you eat per day to maintain a normal weight; sedentary women need to eat about 1,600 calories a day

diaphragm breathing – also called diaphragmatic breathing; inhaling slowly through the nose, tightening stomach muscles, and exhaling through the mouth

echocardiogram (eco) – ultrasound of your heart and blood vessels; tells how well your heart is beating

electrocardiogram (ECG) – test that involves electrodes being placed on our chest to record the heart's electrical impluses

140

Words to Know

emergency room – hospital department with staff that specializes in medical emergencies

exercise – systematic movement, such as Jumping Jacks

food portion – amount of food you choose to eat

food serving – measured amount of food based on nutrition data

high-energy walking – walking at a fast pace; also called speed walking

lipids – fatty deposits in the blood

low-dose aspirin – small tablet between 81 and 325 milligrams; also called baby aspirin

mindful walking – being acutely aware of your body and environment

Nordic walking – brisk walking with two poles

overweight – more weight than is considered healthy for your height, build, and age

obese – well above normal weight; 20 pounds or more

pedometer – small meter that tracks the number of steps you take

physical activity – all types of body movement

pulmonary arteries – carry blood from the right side of the heart to your lungs

pulmonary veins – return blood from the lungs to your heart

race walking – walking with the advancing leg straight and at such a fast pace you never lose contact with the ground

support group – a group of individuals with similar life experiences who meet to share them; usually led by a trained facilitator

target weight – the weight you hope to be, a number that should be realistic and suitable for your height, body type, and age

theme walking – walking with a specific purpose in mind, such as bird watching, looking for a specific color, and walking to museums

trauma center – medical center with a larger staff and more diagnostic equipment than an emergency room

ventricles – lower chambers of the heart

vital signs – pulse, blood pressure, temperature, breaths per minute

walking log – written record of your walking, including date, distance, weather conditions; may include medical symptoms

warm up – slow walking and stretching before you walk

weight loss plateau – after losing weight, a time of no weight loss despite physical activity and healthy eating

About the Author

Harriet Hodgson has been a freelance writer for 35+ years, is the author of hundreds of articles, and 32 published books. She holds a BS from Wheelock College in Boston, Massachusetts, and an MA from the University of Minnesota in Minneapolis, Minnesota. After a dozen years in the classroom Hodgson decided to change careers and turned to writing.

Her current work focuses on health/wellness resources and she is a member of the Association of Health Care Journalists.

A popular guest, Hodgson has appeared on more than 170 talk shows, including CBS Radio, and many television networks, including CNN. Her work is cited in *Something About the Author, Contemporary Authors*, **Who's** *Who of American Women, Who's Who in America, Who's Who in the World*, and *The Dictionary of International Biography*.

Hodgson lives in Rochester, MN with her husband, John, and her twin grandchildren. Married for almost 56 years, the couple still holds hands when they are walking. Visit www.harriethodgson.com

and learn more about this busy author and grandmother. Share your comments and ideas by going to her website, clicking on the blog tab at the top right, and posting. You may also send an email to harriethodgson@charter.net.

Also by Harriet Hodgson

- *Help! I'm Raising My Grandkids: Grandparents Adapting to Life's Surprises,* available from Amazon.
- *Happy Again! Your New and Meaningful Life After Loss,* available from WriteLife, Grief Illustrated Press (a Centering Corporation company), and Amazon.
- *The Spiritual Woman: Quotes to Refresh and Sustain Your Soul,* available from Grief Illustrated Press (a Centering Corporation company) and Amazon.
- *101 Affirmations to Ease Your Grief Journey: Words of Comfort, Words of Hope,* available from Amazon.
- *Writing to Recover: The Journey from Loss and Grief to a New Life,* available from Centering Corporation and Amazon.
- *Writing to Recover Journal,* available from Centering Corporation and Amazon.
- *Smiling Through Your Tears: Anticipating Grief,* Lois Krahn, MD, co-author, available from Amazon.

- *The Alzheimer's Caregiver: Dealing with the Realities of Dementia,* available from Amazon.
- *Alzheimer's, Finding the Words: A Communication Guide for those Who Care,* available from John Wiley & Sons and Amazon.
- *Smart Aging: Taking Charge of Your Physical and Emotional Health,* available from Amazon.

Index